DATE DUE

APR 23	

DEMCO, INC. 38-2931

Survival
First Aid

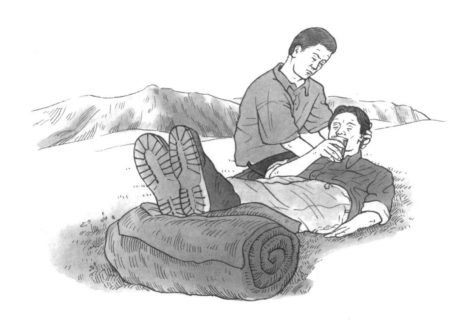

Survival
First Aid

Chris McNab

**CHARTWELL
BOOKS, INC.**

Published by
CHARTWELL BOOKS, INC.
A Division of **BOOK SALES, INC.**
114 Northfield Avenue
Edison, New Jersey 08837

ISBN: 0-7858-1390-X

Editorial and design by
Amber Books Ltd
Bradley's Close
74–77 White Lion Street
London N1 9PF

Design: Hawes Design
Illustrations: Tony Randell and Richard Tibbetts

Neither the author nor the publishers can accept any responsibility for any loss, injury or damage caused as a result of the use of the first aid techniques described in this book, nor for any prosecutions or proceedings brought or instituted against any person or body that may result from using the aforementioned first aid techniques.

Printed in Portugal

Contents

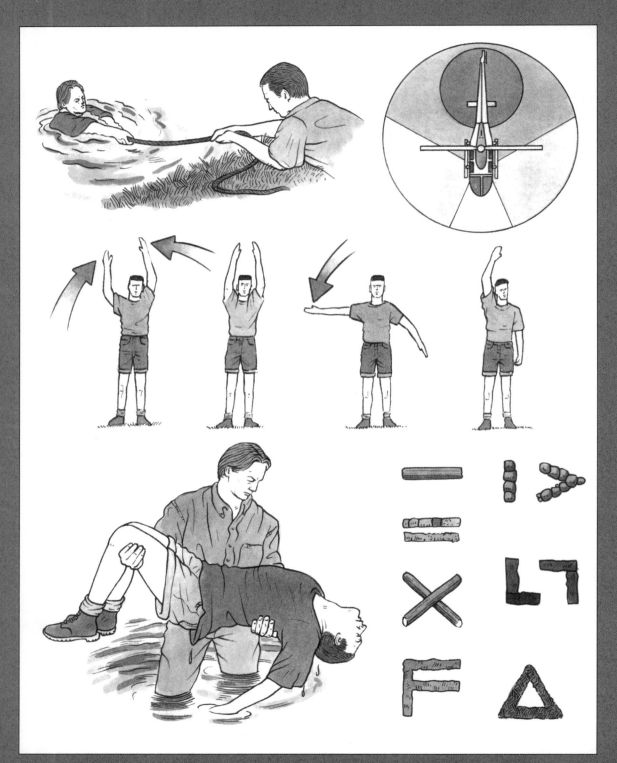

CHAPTER ONE

Preparation & equipment

Survival first aid requires strong nerves, good training and the ability to cope on your own a long way from professional medical help. Exposed to the elements, even the simplest injury can become life-threatening.

Imagine yourself in the following two accident scenarios – in both you are playing the part of a trained first aider. Firstly, you are in a suburban house on the outskirts of a major city. A man has fallen from a high ladder, and you suspect a back injury. The man's tibia (shin bone) has broken, with a sharp end piercing the skin, causing significant blood loss. Symptoms of circulatory shock seem present. The man is drifting in and out of consciousness. Breathing is laboured, and the chest is bruised and swollen. The actual treatment for these conditions will be covered later in the book, but the sequence of your reactions should be: make a diagnosis; protect the patient from any further harm; immediately treat any serious or life-threatening conditions; and, most crucially, contact the emergency services. Because of your

suburban location, the services will often be at your door within minutes of your call, delivering both professional care and transportation to hospital.

For the second situation, transpose the patient to a remote mountain face – he is now the victim of a climbing fall. The injuries are the same; only this time, the demands of your location are very different. You are at least six hours from either a telephone or habitation. Nightfall is only three hours away. The weather has become increasingly worse, with a temperature of −1°C (31°F), worsened by a wind chill factor and slushy rain, which is restricting visibility. There is another member in the party who has no first aid training, and is not as experienced a climber as you. He is suffering from mild altitude sickness. At very best, you would not be able to get the emergency services to your location for another nine hours.

Both examples show the need for positive, controlled action from you as a first aider. Yet the second example also illustrates some of the crucial distinctions between survival first aid in a wilderness context and general first aid. The first aider in the second example must:

- Deliver sustained treatment over a long period without the assistance of professional medical services;
- Be aware of the effect of environmental conditions on the development of the patient's injuries or illness, and on his own ability to deal with them;
- Have a clear system for delivering or attracting a rescue effort from an isolated location without risk to himself or others.

Survival first aid is therefore fundamentally distinguished by its isolation from emergency services, and the unique climatic and environmental conditions which constrain or dictate the treatment the first aider can deliver. This book will explore the practicalities of meeting these unique and demanding circumstances. It will not only present the full range of first aid treatments for all the typical injuries and illnesses first aiders can encounter anywhere, but also those that present themselves in specific environments – ranging from an oxygen-poor mountaintop to a disease-ridden jungle floor.

One word of caution, however, before we go further. If faced with a genuine emergency, it is of paramount importance that any medical procedures you use are based on knowledge rather than the vague desire to do something. Many home-spun ideas about medical treatment are positively dangerous if practised. Using tourniquets to stop bleeding, for instance, will in most situations actually place the casualty in even greater danger (exceptions will be noted later). Giving a

drop of strong alcohol to an unconscious person can make them choke to death. The list goes on and on, from attempting to suck out snake poison to using butter to treat burns. Doing something just for the sake of it can have lethal consequences for your patient, so in all treatments, do what you know will work and nothing more.

- **CAUTION:** As with all first aid books, this manual is intended to act only as a guide to treatment in extreme circumstances. Proper and thorough training should be undertaken before attempting any of these techniques for real. Such courses are especially recommended to those embarking on activities which may involve acute danger or prolonged periods of isolation.

PREPARATION

Some situations in which survival first aid is required are completely unexpected. A car crash on an isolated mountain road, or a ship sinking miles from land, can thrust us from comfort to extremity in a matter of seconds. Much more likely to demand the first aider's skills, however, are accidents or illnesses encountered during outdoor activities in a countryside or wilderness setting. Mountaineering, hiking, mountain biking, pot-holing, canoeing, rafting, sailing, and skiing are just some examples. As sports such as these become increasingly popular, more and more untrained or half-trained individuals are pitting themselves against powerful natural forces far removed from their familiar world. The resulting clash between environment and ignorance generates an increasing need for effective first aid responses.

In reality, first aid awareness should begin before you engage in your chosen activity. Prevention is naturally always better than cure, so it is worth highlighting some of the main considerations in preparing yourself for potentially dangerous outdoor pursuits.

Ideally, these will reduce the possibility of a medical emergency, and help you to cope if one does arise.

Fit to cope

Before launching yourself into remote or exposed places, ask yourself honestly, and everyone else in the group: Are we really fit enough to do this? Embarking on a physically rigorous undertaking, deficient in proper physical resources, not only endangers you but also puts your group at risk should something befall you. In addition, if there are disproportionate levels of fitness within a group, it can easily become disconnected over long distances, with a perilous loss of, or delay in, communication. Thus, you should always engage in a significant period of training which conditions your body specifically for the task in mind. Mix aerobic and anaerobic training in equal measures, and ensure that fitness and strength are both present. If any physical problems come to light during this period of training, you should then question your immediate suitability for any outdoor plans.

A primary caution about physical fitness is to be sensitive to any pre-existing conditions. High or low blood pressure, asthma, angina, diabetes, a previous heart attack, an injury to joints or muscles, epilepsy, even having a cold, flu or swollen lymph nodes, are all preconditions that should make you either think twice about your expedition or journey, or at least make you seek the advice of a doctor before embarking. (In addition, from a legal point of view, undergoing strenuous activity while not being fit to do so can jeopardize your life or health insurance policies.) If there are any pre-existing conditions in the group, everyone should know which symptoms to look out for should they resurface, and know the most appropriate form of treatment. Also, if you are destined for a cold climate, have your teeth checked before you go – dental problems can be severely

exacerbated in persistent low temperatures. Finally, as it is usually feet which bear the brunt of the punishment, make sure they are conditioned before setting out, are well adjusted to the boots you will wear. This is because blisters are not a serious problem if you are returning home at night to a comfortable bath, but if you are spending many days away from domestic hygiene, they can lead to substantial infections and inflammation. So make sure your feet are strong enough to take the pressure.

A close second priority is mental fitness – do you have the experience and knowledge to conduct the enterprise which you intend? If you are going on a mountaineering expedition to a region of Tibet, it will not be enough to have an experience of the mountains in, for example, the US Rockies. Climatic, geographical, social, infrastructural, and medical facilities vary enormously from country to country, and it is imperative that you either gain the knowledge before you go (and do all the relevant preparation) or more preferably, that you go with someone who already possesses the knowledge. The issues with each exploration are very broad, but for first aid awareness the most typical questions you should ask before departure are:

● Are there any distinct climatic/environmental events taking place at the time I am due to visit, for example monsoon, ice melt, tornadoes;
● What health issues should I be aware of? Do I need particular vaccinations? (Typically for illnesses such as hepatitis, smallpox, typhoid, yellow fever, cholera, tuberculosis, diphtheria, and tetanus. Take good stocks of anti-malaria tablets if the region demands it.)
● How well do I know the geography of my destination? You should not only have an acute sense of where you are, but also what types of flora and fauna you might

encounter, where clean water sources are located across the route of travel (and if the water may have unusual natural/chemical contaminants), what type of surfaces you will be crossing, the patterns of sunrise/set, and the most extreme possibilities for daytime/night-time temperatures.

● Are there any social features of which I should be aware? Take advice before travelling around any particularly dangerous areas of the country, what customs you should follow to avoid alienating the locals, and if there are any political/social upheavals which might be impending. Explorers are notoriously vulnerable to hijack, mugging, and even, in certain regions, killing in countries with very low levels of income, so be aware of your areas of travel.

This list is far from exhaustive, and you and the group should meticulously go through any hazards which may arise at your destination. Once you have done this you can go on to plan your expedition. Plan it in great detail, with a rigorous timetable and route plan which are also in the possession of a third party. This third party should have the ability to check on your progress and pick up on any aberrations. Ideally, radio contact is the best safety net, but at the very least have a date or time agreed by which the third party should start to take action to discover your whereabouts. Agree with them on when they should launch a rescue effort – for example, if three attempts to make radio contact over a period of 24 hours have met with no response. Finally, make sure that each member in your group has a specific role to fulfil to avoid confusion in an emergency. Someone should be in overall charge of first aid, including collecting together the relevant items for the first aid kit. Make sure that person submits a checklist of items packed which another person confirms.

EQUIPMENT

The subject of which equipment to take for each specific activity or expedition is mostly beyond the remit of this book, yet there are items which are essential for physical protection and the enhancement of first aid resources. The contents of your medical kit is illustrated in the Appendix on page 190.

Clothing

Clothing is adapted to circumstances, but the overall criteria in selection is that it should supply you with the right levels of warmth and protection, while allowing the skin to breath or 'wick' away perspiration. Your boots (never trainers) should be suited to use, but bear in mind that most boots cannot guarantee waterproofing, so take waterproof liners if appropriate to protect against the dangers of trench foot and fungal infections. Treat the boot leather or fabric regularly, and remember to clean the inside of the boot – regular maintenance inside helps prevent the build up of salts which can contribute to blister formation. (Another blister prevention procedure is to change your socks regularly during the journey itself to avoid rubbing.) When purchasing boots, dual density soles can be a valuable feature for reducing the shock, heavy walking places on knee and ankle joints. Be aware that boots have a sloping front section to the heel may lose grip on wet grass or snow, and the sloping back sections can deprive you of relevant grip on inclines.

For clothing, always avoid cotton as this traps-in water. Many climbers have come unstuck by wearing excellent professional clothing over a common T-shirt which becomes soaked with sweat and then freezes, increasing the danger of hypothermia. All clothes should be able to wick away sweat, and the market has many such items of 'breathable' fabrics available. In hot climates, this may simply mean shirt and shorts of the appropriate material, though be prepared for cold nights, heavy rain, and the possibility of insect attack, when covering up is advisable. Purchase items that give you a high degree of protection from sunburn, as some shirts can allow the easy passage of damaging ultraviolet rays. For temperate and cold climates, clothes should be layered up, the topmost jacket being of a material such as Gore-Tex which allows the skin to disperse sweat droplets while remaining waterproof and windproof, both vital in the protection against hypothermia. Do not just travel in just a fleece – these can quickly become soaked, and generally have few windproof properties (new wind and waterproof fleeces are on the market, but they are very expensive).

Make sure that you have the ability to keep spare clothes dry in your pack should you get wet, as any wet clothes can quickly accelerate the processes of heat loss in cold areas. Of course, another essential for preserving warmth is your sleeping bag. Purchase the best you possibly can, preferably one of the waterproof survival bags to keep you insulated should your tent be lost. Thin silver foil insulation blankets can also be a good idea to take, as they pack up very small and can be used for convenient treatment of patients with heat loss.

Safety equipment

Many survival emergencies have been caused by a simple lack of the most basic survival tools. Make sure that you carry a map and compass (and know how to use them!), and take a method of lighting a fire other than matches – a mountaineer's flint is ideal. Water purification tablets and insect repellent are also essential parts of disease and illness prevention in many countries.

Remember, it is very important to class any untreated water as dangerous, no matter how pure it looks (if a water source has dead animals in the vicinity, you must avoid it completely).

For conditions where you might well encounter snow and ice, an ice axe and crampons are invaluable, but give yourself some good training in the use of these before using them for real to avoid accidental injury though misuse. Even when going on a simple hike, take a climber's safety rope with you and a couple of karabiners each. This rope can be used for everything from negotiating rivers to linking up a group to avoid separation in bad weather. Learn also how to tie a basic figure-of-eight knot (see illustration) to give solid anchorage to karabiners and other anchors. You might also consider taking walking poles with you (note that professionals consider them essential). Using two walking poles can relieve many tons of pressure off your legs for each hour of walking, thus reducing your chances of fatigue injuries in the lower limbs.

Should disaster strike in remote locations, your chances of survival are greatly improved if you have modern means of attracting attention. A strobe light and flares are inexpensive additions to your pack, as is a whistle to provide an auditory locator. And however much you might want to 'get away

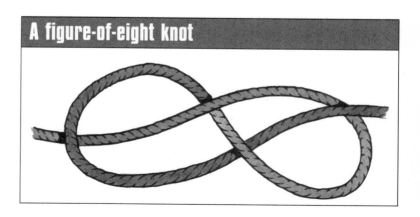

A figure-of-eight knot

Communication essentials

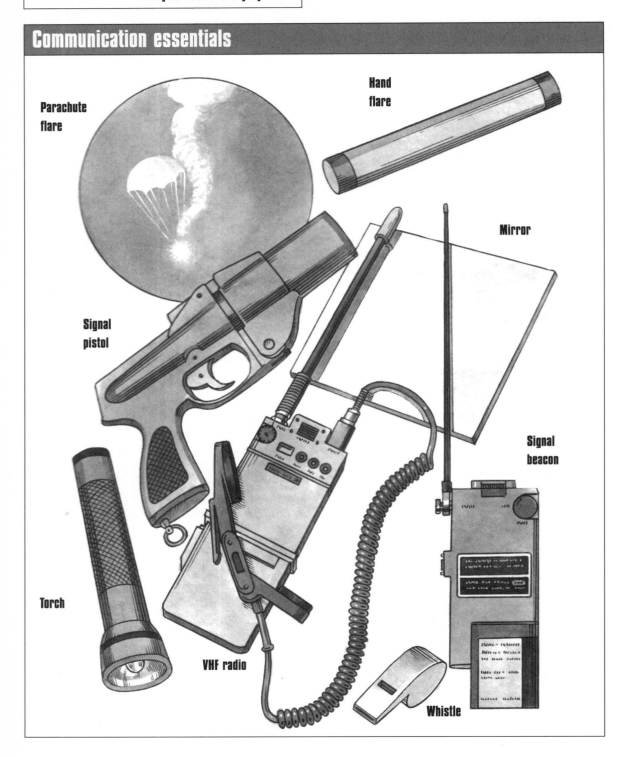

Parachute flare

Hand flare

Mirror

Signal pistol

Signal beacon

Torch

VHF radio

Whistle

from it all', a mobile phone can be a life-saver owing to its ability to achieve a signal from most places in the world (though for certain expeditions, make sure that you have more sophisticated and durable radio and satellite communications).

Finally, when selecting helmets and other safety equipment (especially for climbing), always look for trading standards marks to show that the products conform to international safety standards. The IAA mark is one of the most prevalent and authoritative, but each country will usually have its own product standard system.

Food and nutrition

In addition to the safety items you carry, you should also pay careful attention to the foodstuffs you take with you to eat. Good nutrition is especially important when you are operating at maximum exertion. Make sure that your calorie intake is kept high, and also that your foodstuffs give you the entire range of vitamins, minerals, proteins, carbohydrates, fats, and sugars (the last two are particularly important if you will be in a cold climate). By having a balanced diet your energy levels should be optimal, and you will be able to operate at both your mental and physical best.

IN AN EMERGENCY

Any emergency situation which involves human injury is physically and emotionally chaotic. The sights, sounds, and smells involved can all be shocking, unfamiliar, and disturbing, and, if you allow them to can force you into a mental impotence that deprives you of the ability to act decisively. To function effectively as a first aider in these situations, you must have a fixed pattern of response that is easily followed in the confusion of an emergency. Subsequent chapters will focus on the details of actual medical response, but in this chapter we will examine the practicalities that will govern

your handling of the complete situation – from diagnosis to rescue.

Safety first

Absolutely your first priority in any emergency situation is the safety of yourself and your patient. At any accident site quickly scan around for any dangers-in-waiting. This could mean looking out for further rockfalls or avalanches, or checking that the injured climber to which you are attached is not about to drag you into a fall. Particular danger is possible if you can smell gas or petrol, and you should beware of possible sources of electrical or combustible ignition (switch off any vehicle ignition). If a fire is present, and it is safe to do so, remove any explosive or inflammable materials such as flares, gas canisters, ammunition, or oxygen cylinders from the vicinity, and make sure that all tents in an area are empty and all people accounted for.

As you are mostly likely to be in an area without large-scale artificial lighting, do not attempt any precarious rescue or medical treatment at night without adequate illumination from a torch or other source, and have another person direct the illumination, leaving your hands free to work. Helmet torches can give you the best of both worlds.

One of the additional strains of being a survival first aider is that your environment makes it far more likely that you will have to actually rescue your patient before you can apply first aid. It would be impossible to be prescriptive about the specifics of a rescue attempt, but there are some general rules which apply to certain situations.

Fire

Fires are less common in outdoor situations than in household settings, but can occur with the use of cooking equipment within or around tents (make sure that the tents you use are made of fire retardant material). If a person is on fire, try to stop the patient running

Vehicle rescue procedure

Observe the vehicle in which the patient is trapped at a distance (unless you are actually in the vehicle) to see any signs of petrol leakage, fire, electrical sparks, or dangerous contents (particularly extra petrol cans often stored in wilderness exploration vehicles). Remember to shed any metal implements you are carrying to avoid the risk of sparking an ignition. If there are no immediate signs of danger, advance to the vehicle, switch off the ignition even if the engine has stopped, disconnect the battery if possible, and proceed to treat the patient. Vehicles such as diesel vans, trucks, and buses and motorcycles often have the means available to disconnect their fuel supply. As a rule, if the casualty cannot walk away from the vehicle you should initially treat them in it.

However, if the car does seem to be in danger of ignition, remove the patient as quickly as possible, smashing the glass if doors are jammed shut.

● *NOTE:* only move the patient if the danger to them from fire or explosion is greater than that of aggravating a possible spinal injury.

If a vehicle has crashed on a steep or mountainous road, ensure that its hand brake is on, and that large stones are placed under its wheels (even if the tyres are punctured) to prevent it running away.

around and thus fanning the flames, drop them to the ground and then either a) roll the patient on the ground until flames are smothered; b) wrap them in a heavy non-flammable material (not nylon); or c) douse them in water or other non-flammable liquid.

Drowning

The first principle of rescuing a drowning person is not to go in after them if they are beyond standing-depth water, and if you are not properly trained in water-environment rescue techniques. A drowning person usually goes into a blind panic, and if you are in the water with them, they will attempt to climb on top of you or even fight you in their hysteria. As this can drag you down with them, it is far better to stay on the bank and to throw them some form of buoyancy aid. If they are close to the bank, offer them a long stick or toss them the end of a rope.

If you really have to enter the water and swim out to the victim, take some sort of buoyancy aid with you, and relinquish it to the drowning person (as long as you can swim back to bank) or share it with them. Try to calm the person as much as possible to make them cooperative in the rescue.

Avalanche

After only one hour buried underneath an avalanche, a person's life expectancy is reduced by about 50 per cent, so quick action by those in the vicinity is imperative. Keep on the lookout for further avalanche danger, but note the last position at which the missing person was seen.

Search from that point downward, looking for any items of clothing or equipment and listening carefully for any cries. Leave the found items where they are so that you have a clear idea of the person's fall trajectory through the avalanche. If the victim is found, quickly dig them out, clear their airway of any snow or ice and treat, if necessary, for hypothermia (see page 149). If they are not found after an hour, go quickly for expert help.

NOTE: the use of connecting ropes and transceivers greatly simplify the detection of victims.

Infections

Remember that the patient himself, and not only your environment, could be one of your greatest dangers. Blood- or fluid-borne diseases are a serious threat if you are to come into contact with any person suffering from a bleeding injury, or one who requires mouth-to-mouth resuscitation. The main dangers are hepatitis A, B and (less commonly) C, D, and G, and HIV (the virus which leads to AIDS), and in certain developing countries you may also encounter other infectious illnesses such as tuberculosis and typhoid.

In a first aid context, hepatitis and HIV infection would mainly be through blood-to-blood contact between the injured party and the first aider. So pack your medical kit with latex medical gloves to avoid blood and skin contact, wear eye protectors to shield against blood splashes, wash yourself thoroughly after treating the patient, and dispose of all soiled materials safely after use. If you have to give mouth-to-mouth resuscitation, use a face shield (if you have one) which fits over the patient's face and allows you to give Cardio-Pulmonary Resuscitation (CPR) without skin-to-skin contact (see Chapter Three).

As unpleasant a task as it may be, exercise diligence in clearing away all bodily waste which your patient produces. Blood, vomit, and excreta will all attract flies, disease, and encourage infections, so safely transfer them away from the area of treatment. Bury or burn if possible.

● **NOTE:** In countries which suffer from poor sanitation, your medical pack should contain sterilized hypodermic syringes and scalpel blades. These are not only for you to use on your patient, but they can also be given to the indigenous medical staff to protect against diseases transferred through infected medical equipment.

TAKING CONTROL

Your first reaction when faced by an emergency situation may well be one of psychological shock. The demands of the situation

Rope rescue

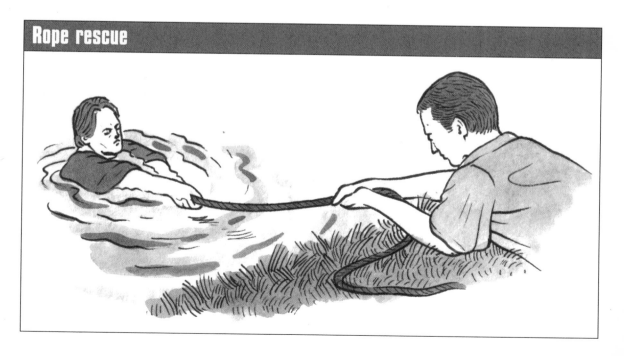

'Head back' carrying technique for drowning victim

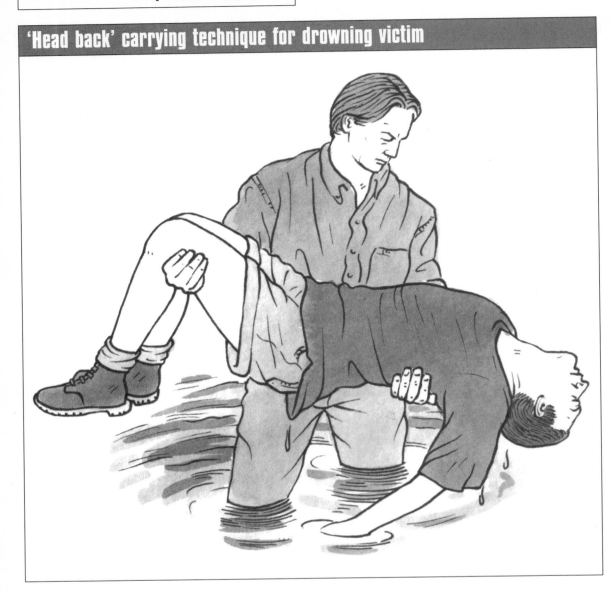

will release hormones, adrenaline, noradrenaline, and cortisol into the bloodstream which give the body dramatic power, but which can also stop a person acting with the clear and steady thinking essential for the delivery of effective first aid.

Your first response should be to take deep, calming breaths, and to begin to assess the situation rationally, however traumatic it might appear. When you have calmed yourself and made an initial assessment, follow this step-by-step procedure:

● Assess the situation, work out if there are any new dangers present, and establish who has been injured. If there are two or more of you still physically capable, put one in charge of the situation to avoid a confusion of efforts. Ideally, the person with the most first aid training should be in control. Then follow the DATE system with each casualty:

- **Diagnosis** - Evaluate the nature of the patient's illness or injuries.
- **Assessment** - Work out the most appropriate form of first aid treatment.
- **Treatment** - Deliver and maintain that treatment.
- **Evacuation** - Ensure that the patient is evacuated to a professional medical centre as quickly as possible.

Work through each of these procedures, one step at a time, using the treatment methods given in this book or in any other good first aid manual. In all of these steps, however, know your own limitations. Do not deliver any treatments about which you are not confident. If there are multiple casualties, you may have to make some hard choices about whom to treat. A good guideline is to first go to those casualties who are silent – even if a person is screaming violently, it suggests that for the time-being their airway is clear and they are conscious. Once you have made your choice on sound reasons then stick with it until the situation changes. Remember you can only be in one place at once, and saving one life is better than losing two. If you can, enlist people to help you. Some first aid procedures can be exhausting, so split burdens if possible to make your efforts more effective.

Giving confidence

Underlying all your dealings with the casualties should be an attempt to make them as calm as possible, thus reducing the impact that psychological shock is making upon their situation. Always talk quietly but confidently, and let the patient feel reassured by your presence. Some points to bear in mind are:

- Try to shield the patient from distressing sights of other persons injured or killed. Encourage them to look only at you and if possible use others' equipment (such as a pack) to limit the patient's view.
- Always remember that of all the human senses, hearing is usually the last sense to fail in the human being. Even patients in a deep coma have shown through brain scans that they have some level of response to what is being said around them. So even if the patient appears deeply unconscious, keep talking to them in the usual reassuring manner. Be especially aware of other people around you who may not know this. Someone asking 'Is he dead?' may achieve just that result by the shock they induce, so signal to people to be quiet as they approach.
- Use your judgement as to how to answer the patient's questions. Try not to reveal too much detail if the patient's injuries are severe, but keep the focus on the positive actions that you are taking, and on the positive things the patient can do to make the situation better.

GETTING HELP

Never forget that there is always a limit to what you can achieve with first aid. First aid is essentially the practice of damage limitation, not complete cure. In an emergency, always keep your mind fastened on the end result, which is to get a seriously ill or injured person into the hands of medical professionals within the facilities of a modern hospital or clinic.

Of course, in a survival situation that is much easier said than done. Even the process of contacting the emergency services can be a hazardous and complicated procedure when you are many miles from civilization. The practicalities of bringing in an outside rescue force should have been discussed or arranged in detail *prior* to leaving on your journey or expedition. Moreover, if you are travelling to somewhere especially remote you should take with you the necessary communication equipment to make on-location contact possible. If you are using VHF radios or other types of transmitters, test them thoroughly before setting out, making sure that their batteries have power for the entire trip.

Yet when technological communications are not available or fail, you must fall back on a physical method of attracting rescue. Any rescue attempt begins with the attempt to let outside parties know where you are, and the type of trouble you are in. This means that you either communicate from where you are using, various artificial means, or that you physically go and find help.

Travelling for help

The golden rule in any survival situation is not to break up your party unless you are under the most pressing emergency. In the context of first aid, this would mean that your patient is in life-threatening danger from his injuries or illness, and which can only be handled by professional personnel away from the scene of the accident.

Your approach to going and seeking help depends on the size and nature of the party. Firstly, decide who is most appropriate to go. If you are in an area of especially difficult terrain, the likeliest candidate is the person who has experience in dealing with that terrain. They will be able to travel much more quickly than anyone else, with the least danger of incurring injury. Also, the person with the highest level of first aid training should stay with the casualty.

Naturally, the situation in which you find yourself will alter with the dynamics of both who is injured and the medical and environmental prognosis. However, the need to get help illustrates why you should always go exploring in teams of three or more, but be careful about groups of over 10 people, which can become unwieldy and uncoordinated. If your party is a sizeable one (i.e. over four), send out two people to get help, but make sure that they are co-ordinated in both their intentions and in the information they intend to present to the rescue authorities.

One of the most awkward situations is deciding whether to go for help when you are simply one of a couple. Your decision will be based on a delicate judgement about whether you serve your injured partner better by staying or going. Usually it is best to stay and take care of him, especially if he is unconscious. Either wait for a spontaneous rescue attempt to come to you, or try to attract attention to yourself using whatever means available (see 'Signalling for help' on page 21). If you are unlikely to be discovered, then try to place your partner in a sheltered spot (or build a shelter), make sure he is warm and waterproof, leave a note on him explaining his condition, and then set off for help. Before you do so, mark his location with anything conspicuous so that you can direct your rescuers to him – Day-Glo clothing is ideal

Whatever your situation, if it is you that has been chosen to go for help, you should adopt the following procedure:

- Note down the details of your situation, as fatigue may weaken your memory by the time you get to help. Note your location, the name of the natural feature, map location, compass points, prominent landmarks, full details of the type of injuries present, whether the injured person has any special medical history (for example, diabetes). Write down the time of the accident and the time at which you leave for help. This information will be vital to guide the emergency services' rescue efforts.

- Have a clear idea of where you are going and the time it will take for you to summon rescue. Over- rather than under-estimate this time scale (double it is a good

Morse code

A .▬	M ▬▬	Y ▬.▬▬
B ▬...	N ▬.	Z ▬▬.. ▬
C ▬.▬.	O ▬▬▬	1 .▬▬▬▬
D ▬..	P .▬▬.	2 ..▬▬▬
E .	Q ▬▬.▬	3 ...▬▬
F ..▬.	R .▬.	4 ....▬
G ▬▬.	S ...	5 .....
H	T ▬	6 ▬....
I ..	U ..▬	7 ▬▬...
J .▬▬▬	V ...▬	8 ▬▬▬..
K ▬.▬	W .▬▬	9 ▬▬▬▬.
L .▬..	X ▬..▬	0 ▬▬▬▬▬

Ground signals

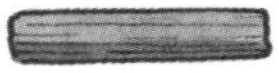

Doctor needed

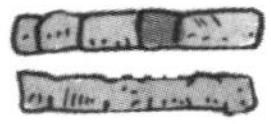

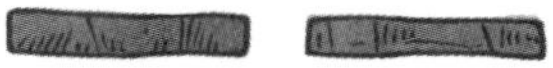

Signal lamp and radio needed

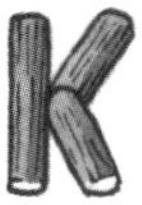

L

Food and oil needed

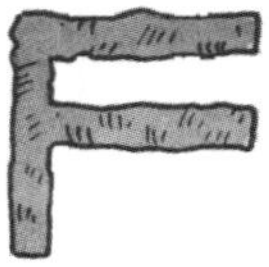

Medical supplies needed

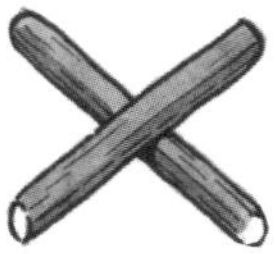

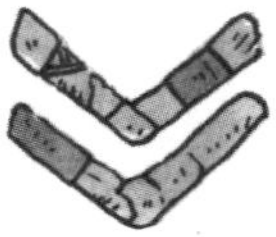

K

Indicate which direction to follow

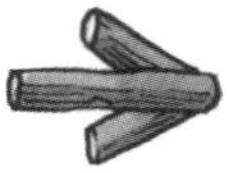

LL

Everything OK

X

Unable to proceed

Moving in this direction

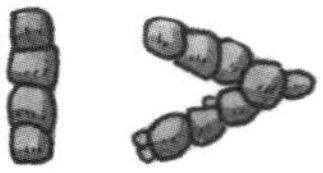

N

No

F

Food and water needed

Will attempt take-off

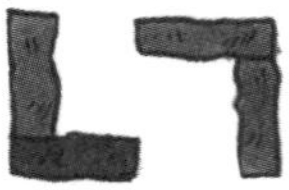

Y

Yes

Firearms needed

Aircraft damaged

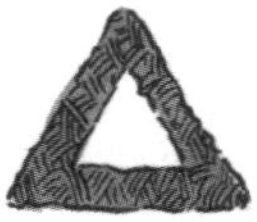

JL

Not understood

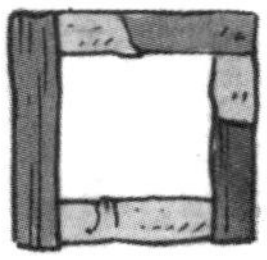

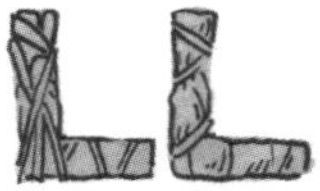

Map and compass needed

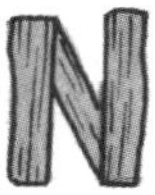

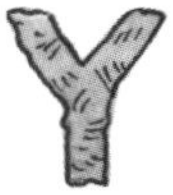

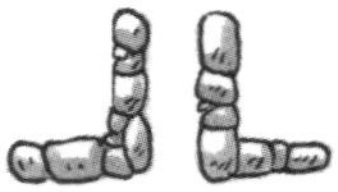

Safe to land here

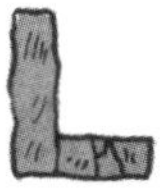

W

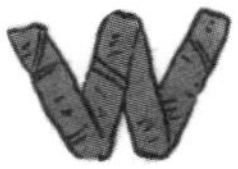

Engineer needed

guide), and let the rest of your party know so that if you or rescuers do not reach them by a certain time, then the remainder can start their own rescue proceedings.

● Set out for rescue, making a good note of the route of your journey. Always maintain a sense of who or what you are trying to reach (usually a communication point or a point of habitation). If you are in an especially remote part of the world, make sure that you have enough provisions with you for the undertaking.

● Once you have made contact with professional (or otherwise) emergency services, give them your location and the patient's location. Unless otherwise instructed, stay where you are so that the rescue services can pick you up and use you to direct them to the right spot. Give them all the information you have jotted down so that they are properly equipped to deal with the emergency once they get there. Remember, if you are hunting for a telephone to call emergency services, make sure you know a) the right number for the country you are in; and b) that you have the means to communicate with the person you have contacted if they speak another language (learn key words and phrases before you go).

If you achieve all these steps, then the rescue should effectively be out of your hands. However, those who have remained with the patient will still have responsibilities for signalling their location and presence to the rescue unit, particularly in large wilderness areas or where weather is poor. Also they may have to direct the operation in a helicopter rescue. The techniques of helicopter rescue are treated in the box opposite.

SIGNALLING FOR HELP

There are two main methods of signalling: visual or auditory. Auditory options are fairly limited. Blowing a whistle and shouting as load as possible can attract attention, depending on wind direction, acoustics, and noise interference, up to half a mile away. If there are two of you shouting, try to shout at different pitches. This creates a stronger sound pattern and increases your likelihood of being heard. If you use a whistle, follow the international distress signal of six long bursts of noise every minute. This signal pattern also applies to visual signalling when using a torch or other controllable medium.

It is, however, the visual field which gives the most varied opportunities for gaining contact. We will explore the main options here.

Fire

A fire can be an excellent identifier, especially in densely wooded areas. Remember that during the day you are aiming for a very smoky fire, so keep it fed with green wood boughs, grass, ferns, and any other materials which produce plentiful smoke. In a snowscape, putting oil or rubber on the fire gives the most visible dark smoke patterns, whereas at night, a bright red blazing fire is best. Three fires set in a triangle are an international distress signal, but be ready to light them quickly, and beware causing a forest fire which could further endanger you.

Light

Light signals can be produced by using a torch or a shining surface which reflects sunlight. A mirror is ideal for this latter function, but if this is not available, then use any metal object polished as bright as possible.

International rescue codes

● **SOS**
Pyrotechnics: Red flare
Auditory signal: 3 short, 3 long, 3 short – repeat every minute
Light flashes: 3 short, 3 long, 3 short – repeat every minute

● **HELP NEEDED**
Pyrotechnics: Red flare
Auditory signal: 6 blasts in quick succession – repeat every minute
Light flashes: 6 flashes in quick succession – repeat every minute

● **MESSAGE UNDERSTOOD**
Pyrotechnics: Red flare
Auditory signal: 3 blasts in quick succession – repeat every minute
Light flashes: 3 flashes in quick succession – repeat every minute

● **RETURN TO BASE**
Pyrotechnics: Green flare
Auditory signal: Quick succession of sustained blasts
Light flashes: Quick succession of sustained flashes

21

Body signals

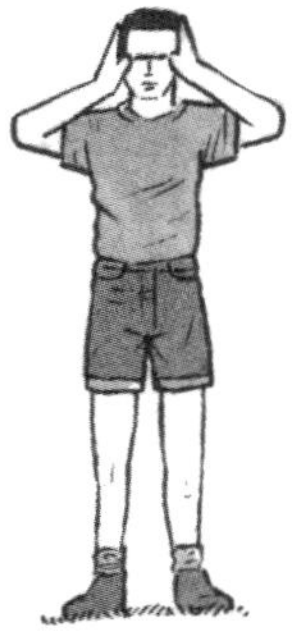

Our receiver is operating

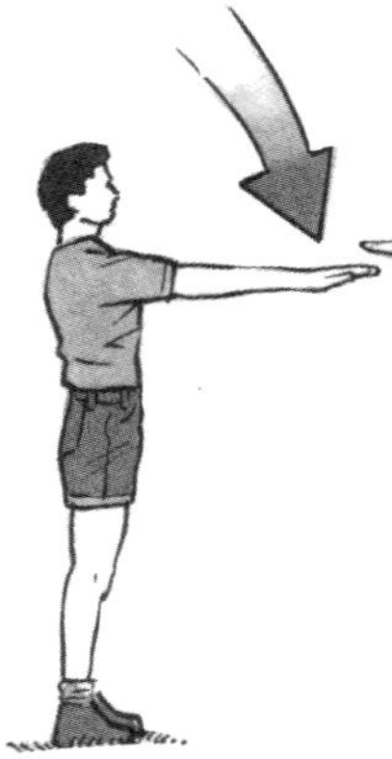

Yes

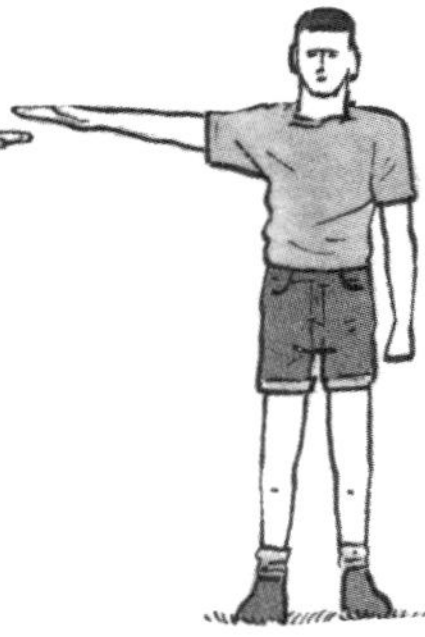

Can move soon, wait if possible

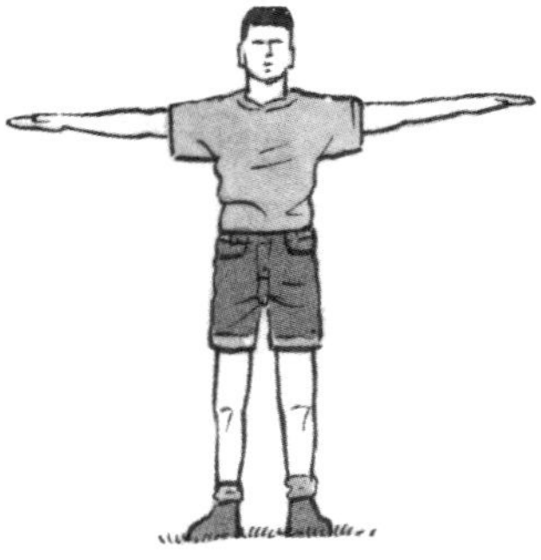

Mechanical help needed long delay

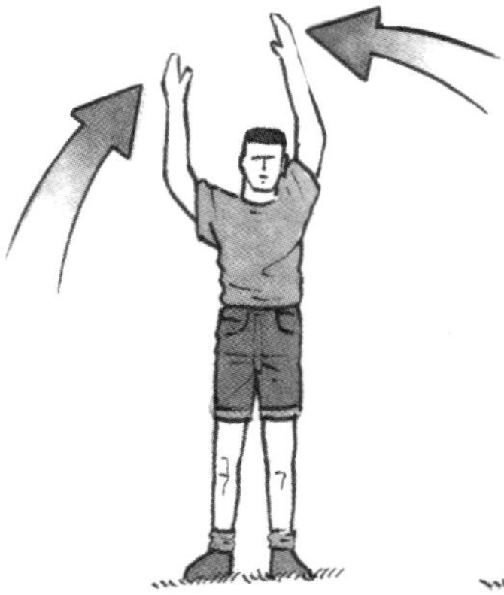

Do not land here

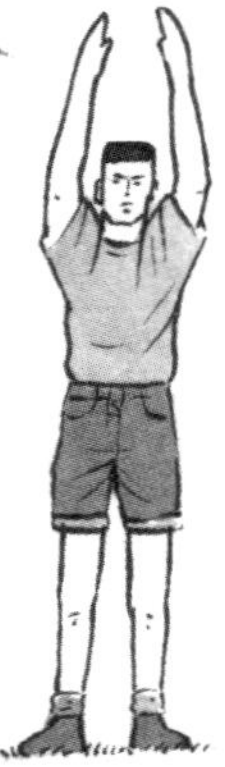

Pick us up

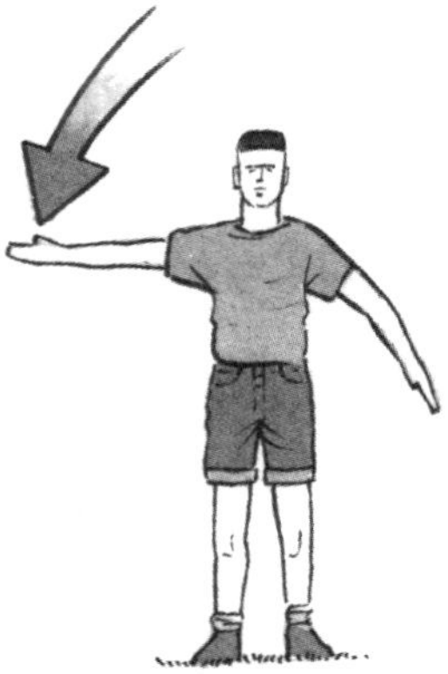

Drop a message

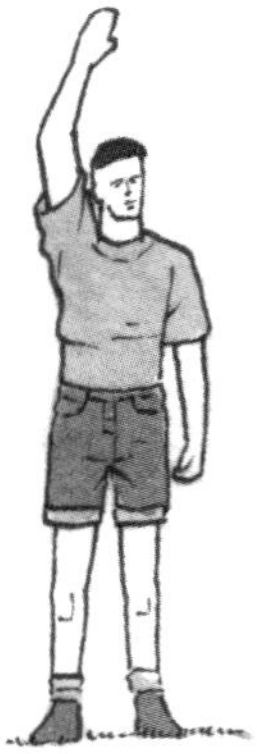

Everything OK – do not wait

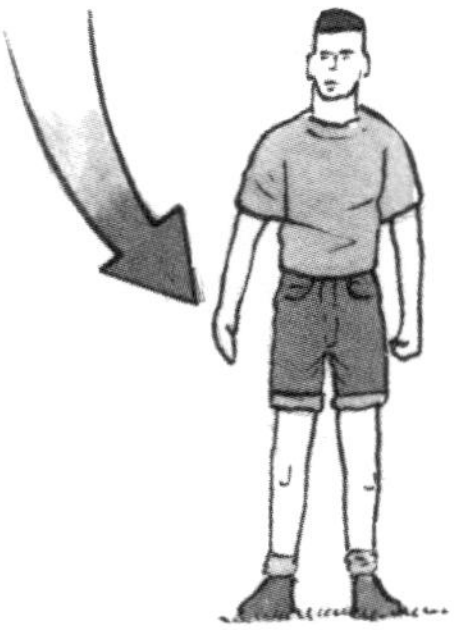

No

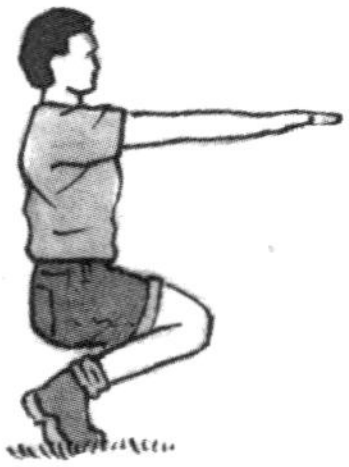

Land here (pointing)

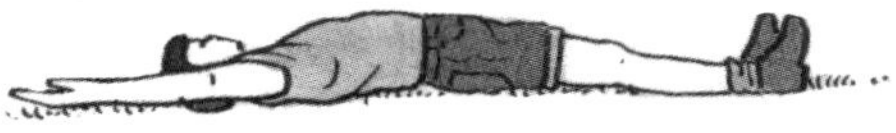

Urgent medical assistance required

Ground-to-air signals

There is an internationally recognized group of marking signals with which you should be familiar before you set out on your journey (see page 20), and you should also carry purpose-designed marker panels which can be obtained from any professional supplier. Lay these signals out in exposed places using prominent materials, preferably in bright colours. If you have none, improvise using whatever natural and man-made materials come to hand, but make them bold enough to be seen at distance – 10m (32.8ft) in length is recommended. If your signals attract attention and a return signal, respond in return with the appropriate message.

A ground-to-air signal can also be made in snow by heaping it up into the relevant patterns to a height of about 1m (3ft). The resulting shadow effect makes a clear pattern.

Body signals

Remember to make them as clear and bold as possible. Use aids such as brightly coloured pieces of material held or tied to limbs to make each signal as clear as possible.

Pyrotechnic signals

Pyrotechnic signals are especially prominent, but you must ensure that you know exactly how to use them before leaving on your journey. Serious burns occur through misuse. Flares vary in type from smoke, parachute, and pistol-launched flares, to the 'bird-scarer' type which explode with a load aerial bang. Use the flares appropriate to your circumstances, and do not waste them in panic. Choose a colour of flare most suited to the background against which it is fired.

Flares should be used with the correct etiquette (see page 21) but again, learn this before you go!

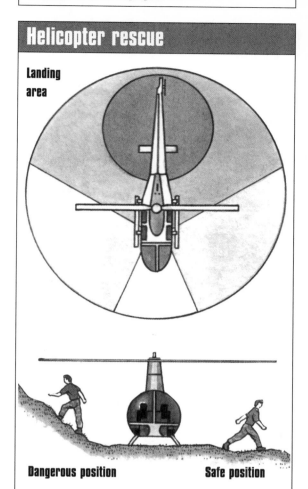

Helicopter rescue

Landing area

Dangerous position   Safe position

Helicopter rescue etiquette varies according to the situation. If the helicopter will land, be situated at a flat area over 25m (82ft), which has freedom of approach with take-off routes into the prevailing winds. Flatten or remove any objects which conflict with the landing. Indicate wind speed and direction to the pilot by setting off a smoke flare away from the landing site and downwind, or tie a piece of coloured material to a tree as a wind sock. When the helicopter lands, approach from the side at a crouch (never from a downward sloping position which may take you close to the blades), and allow the winchman to direct your entry.

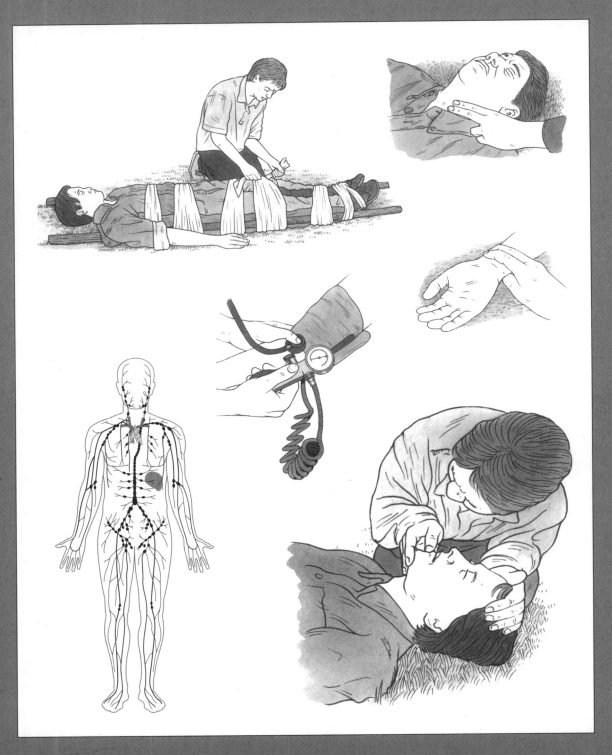

CHAPTER TWO

The human body & first aid

The human physique is both incredibly strong and intensely vulnerable. Life is sustained around the efficient functioning of three major body systems – circulatory, respiratory and nervous – and knowing how they work forms the basis of much of your emergency first aid treatment.

First aid is primarily about immediate and practical treatments, so advanced medical knowledge is not a pre-requisite. However, it is advantageous if the first aider comprehends the biological cornerstones of human life, for without an understanding of the body's basic mechanisms, it is difficult to adapt treatments to meet unexpected developments in the illness or injury. Furthermore, without understanding or appreciating the reason for your actions, it can be more difficult to best apply yourself.

We begin this chapter with a look at the three biological systems responsible for maintaining human life – the respiratory, circulatory, and nervous systems. From there, we move onto the fundamentals of first aid practice – diagnosis, assessment, and treatments when one or more of the major body systems is in acute failure.

THE BODY'S SYSTEMS

For a first aider, the essential principle to remember is that the oxygenation of the

The respiratory system

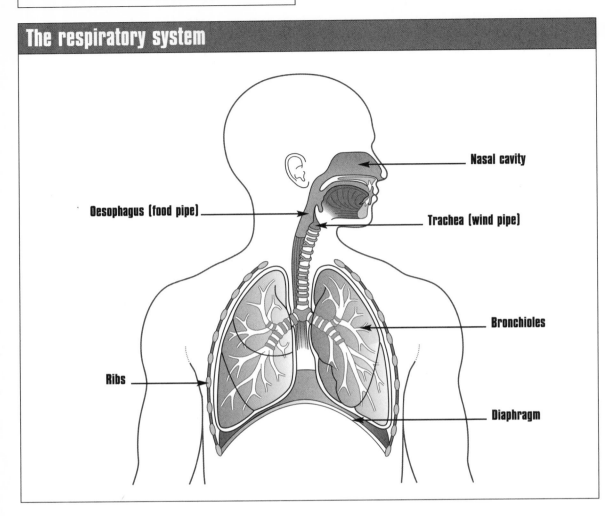

Nasal cavity

Oesophagus (food pipe)

Trachea (wind pipe)

Bronchioles

Ribs

Diaphragm

human body must be maintained at all times. All human tissue, but especially the major organs of the body, will quickly die if deprived of oxygen. It is the respiratory system's job to draw air from the outside world, extract the oxygen and pass it into the blood. It is the job of the circulatory system to pump this blood around the body, and deliver oxygen to the body tissue while extracting waste products. Finally, the nervous system regulates the pace and efficiency of the whole process.

When a first aider is faced with a casualty, their attention is (initially) totally given over to supporting the efficient function of all three systems if need be. For if any system fails, the result is hypoxia, or low levels of blood-borne oxygen. For example, a patient has an obstructed windpipe, then the respiratory system cannot draw air into the lungs, and the blood receives no new oxygen. This in turn means that the circulatory system does not contain enough oxygen in the blood to perform full-body oxygenation properly (a condition known as ischemia).

Hypoxia, if not corrected, leads to infarction, the death of body tissue and organs. The brain is one of the most vulnerable organs to ischemic problems. Brain cells begin to die after only three minutes of deprivation, and if completely deprived of oxygen for more than five minutes, brain damage or brain death will almost certainly ensue. Consequently, in life-threatening emergencies the combating of ischemia is the first aider's absolute priority. That involves the effective support of all three body systems, and we shall now look at each in more detail.

Respiratory System

The respiratory system consists of the mouth, nose, trachea, and lungs, and includes the network of pulmonary arteries that take oxygen from the lungs to the bloodstream. Breathing is controlled by the autonomic nervous system – the part of our brain and nerve network that regulates essential involuntary processes such as the heartbeat and body temperature. All breathing begins with inspiration (breathing in). This occurs when a network of muscles including the intercostal (between the ribs) muscles, the diaphragm, and muscle groups in the abdomen and neck work together to expand the chest cavity, creating a vacuum in the lungs which causes air to rush in via the nose or mouth.

The air passes down the nose and trachea, a cartilage tube of between 10 and 12cm (4–4.75in) in an adult, which then subdivides into the bronchi (the first inverted Y-shape division is known as the stem bronchi). These subdivide continually to form a complete network of air passages in the lungs, and then subdivide even further into bronchioles, minute air passages which each terminate in an alveolus.

The alveoli are millions of microscopic air sacs where the all-important transfer of oxygen into the blood and carbon dioxide out of the blood takes place. Thin-walled blood vessels known as capillaries (pulmonary capillaries in this case) surround each alveolus. Each capillary is tiny in

diameter, and these receive oxygen into the blood stream through the wall of the alveoli, while passing back carbon dioxide and other wastes in the opposite direction. The wastes are vented by the last stage of breathing – expiration. Expiration is achieved when the rib muscles relax, return to position, and push the lung contents out of the nose or mouth.

The average adult breathes at a rate of between 12 and 20 cycles per minute, depending on the level of exertion (greater oxygenation of the body is required to support intensive physical effort). The overall rate is controlled by the brain, which monitors the pH levels in the blood relative to the amount of carbon dioxide present – too much carbon dioxide and respiration is increased to aid its removal.

The problems of the respiratory system will be explored in Chapter Three, but the following are the most common causes of respiratory failure:

- **Airway obstruction** - foreign body stuck in throat; swollen tongue or throat; strangulation; liquid in airpipe.
- **Oxygen deprivation** - smoke or gas inhalation; altitude sickness.
- **Chest or lung injuries** - crushed chest; broken ribs; punctured lung; pneumothorax; haemothorax; internal burns from inhaling super-heated air.
- **Poisoning** - carbon monoxide and other gases (poisoning can reduce the lungs ability to process oxygen).
- **Head injury** - damage to either the part of the brain or the nerves involved in the control of breathing.
- **Secondary impairment** - heart attack or shock resulting in the stoppage of breathing.
- **Allergies and disease** - asthma; anaphylactic shock; bronchitis; pneumonia.
- **Hysterical/psychological** - panic attack; sudden fear.

The circulatory system

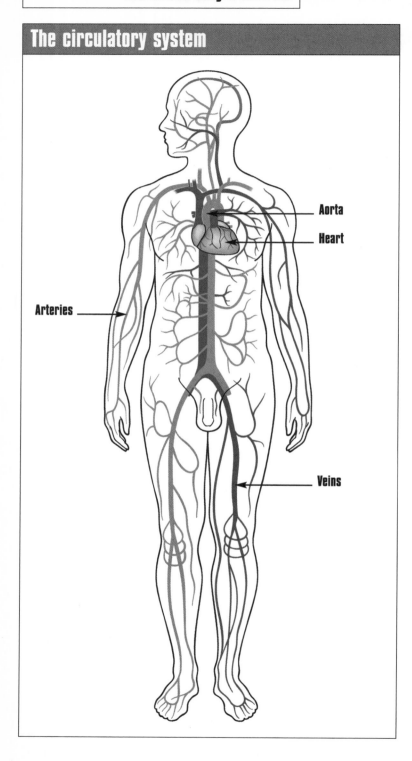

Aorta

Heart

Arteries

Veins

Circulatory System

The circulatory system, like the respiratory, works in a cycle. At the centre of the cycle is the human heart. This immensely durable muscle beats, rhythmically and regularly, to pump oxygenated blood throughout the network of blood vessels in the body. The heart beats at an average resting pace of about 60–90 beats per minute, climbing towards 190 during heavy exertion, when the body's demand for oxygen is at its highest.

The circulatory system starts its cycle when deoxygenated blood flows via the veins into the right chamber of the heart, the atrium, before being pumped out of the right pumping chamber, the ventricle, towards the lungs through the pulmonary artery. The blood is thus oxygenated and returns to the heart, where it collects in the left atrium and is pumped from the left ventricle through the aorta (the body's largest artery) and around the rest of the body. The flow of blood around the body – veins taking blood to the heart and arteries taking it away – is aided by the contractions of the blood vessels themselves, which squeeze the blood on its passage. Between the small veins and arteries are thin-walled capillaries which allow nutrients and oxygen to be passed into body tissue, while also allowing waste products to be removed.

The heart and the blood vessels form the essential circulatory system, but they are part of a much wider physiological organization dedicated to the efficient processing and use of blood. The spleen, liver, kidneys, and urinary system are all involved in the vital cleaning and regulation of blood content. Its involvement with complex major organs makes the circulatory system vulnerable to a significant catalogue of complaints and dangers, but from the first aider's point of view, there is a basic range of injuries or illnesses to be aware of:

- **Shock** – not psychological shock, but the serious physiological shock resulting from blood or fluid loss from the bloodstream (see Chapter Three).
- **Blood vessel damage or impairment** – blood vessels can be damaged by external injury, or blocked by an internal blood clot. Either way, the effect is to stop the effective cycle of blood movement.
- **Reduction in oxygenation** – problems with the patient's breathing eventually impact on the circulatory system as oxygen levels in the blood are lowered. Hypoxia can also result from various forms of anaemia (a reduction in the red blood cells' quantities of haemoglobin, which carries oxygen around the body). Anaemia can occur for many reasons, from blood loss to genetically inherited illnesses (such as sickle-cell anaemia).
- **Impairment of heart function** – the arteries of the heart can go into sudden constriction or be obstructed (such as through a thrombosis), resulting in a heart attack. In this condition, the heart either stops beating or beats rapidly and ineffectively. Another common heart condition is angina, when the heart does not receive enough blood during times of exertion due to narrowed coronary arteries.

Nervous System

The nervous system consists of the central nervous system, peripheral nervous system, and autonomic nervous system.

The central nervous system is the 'engine room' of human nervous response and regulation. It contains the billions of nerve cells which go to make up the brain and the spinal column. We tend to associate the brain with the activities of thought, emotion, and consciousness, but it also has regulatory control over many of the body's vital functions such as breathing and heart rate. Injuries to the brain can impact quickly upon the overall efficiency of human physiology.

The brain is subdivided. The front part of its mass, known as the cerebrum, accounts for some two-thirds of the brain's average 1.4kg (3lb) weight, and is principally responsible for conscious thought, speech, aspects of movement, and the unifying of sensory information. Following this is the cerebellum (situated at the back of the skull, level with the ears), which picks up sensory signals, and generates the appropriate muscular response and controls balance. Finally, there is the brain stem which runs from the centre of the brain down into the spinal column. This is crucially responsible for breathing, blood pressure and consciousness itself. Thus in medical practice, brain stem death is often judged as the final indication that a person's life has truly ceased. The whole of the brain is protected by three membranes, known as the meninges, with the cerebrospinal fluid which provides a cushioning effect between the brain and the skull (the fluid also passes nutrition and oxygen to the brain).

The second part of the central nervous system is the spinal cord, the protection of which features heavily in any first aid manual. This is because the spinal cord is not only responsible for much of human reflex action, but it is also the main conduit by which information from the peripheral nerves is passed to the brain. The cord itself is about 45cm (18in) long, and runs down through the bones of the vertebrae.

After the central nervous system comes the peripheral nervous system. The peripheral nervous system effectively links the sensory information from the muscles, skin, and skeleton to the brain and spinal column. There are three main groupings:

1) The cranial nerves which consist of 12 pairs of nerves going out from the base of the brain, and which report on vital bodily functions from smell to heart beat.

2) The spinal nerves, which pass messages from skin and muscle to the spinal column and back again.

3) A collection of other nerves which contribute to the autonomic nervous system. This last system comprises certain nerves which regulate essential bodily functions such as heart rate, body temperature, physiological motivation and digestion.

The spectrum of responsibility accounted for by the nervous systems means that problems within it can range from a mild headache to an immediate fatality. From a

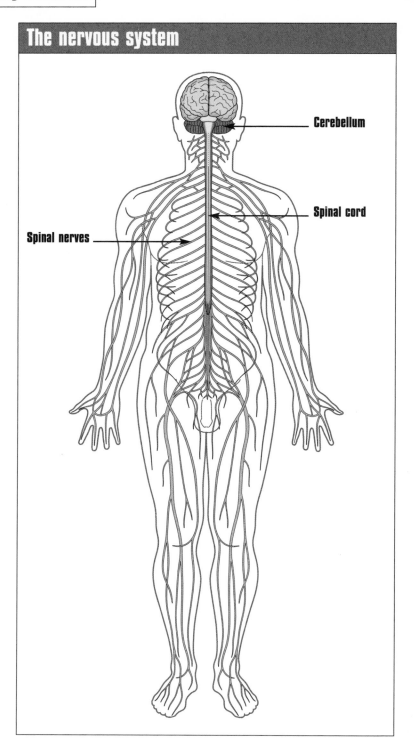

The nervous system

Cerebellum

Spinal cord

Spinal nerves

first aid point of view, the types of problems encountered fall into eight distinct categories, some of them specific to survival environments.

- **Head injury** – An injury to the brain, either through direct damage or compression, such as caused by a fractured skull.
- **Spinal column injury or compression** – damage to the vertebrae of the spine can result in damage to the spinal column itself, with a consequent loss of body sensation or physiological control or different levels of paralysis.
- **Brain infections or diseases** – some illnesses of the brain, such as multiple sclerosis or Parkinson's disease, are unlikely to be encountered in survival situations owing to their steadily degenerative nature. Others, however, like meningitis or the sudden eruption of an unknown brain tumour, can strike at any time.
- **Stroke** – though mostly, but not exclusively, an affliction of old age, one in four of us will suffer or die from a stroke. It is caused by the haemorrhaging or blockage of a blood vessel in the brain which restricts the brain's circulation and oxygen levels.
- **Blood sugar imbalance** – dangerously low or dangerously high blood sugar levels, known as hypoglycaemia and hyperglycaemia respectively, can both lead to loss of consciousness and even coma. These conditions are mostly associated with diabetes.
- **Epilepsy** – epilepsy stems from the disruption of the electrical patterns within the brain, and is used as a generic term to cover a wide manner of convulsions and fits. These range from 'grand mal' seizures, in which there is a complete loss of consciousness, through to 'petit mal' or focal seizures which afflict only certain parts of the body, with momentary periods of awareness.

The list of afflictions given here for the circulatory, nervous, and respiratory systems will be explored in greater depth in the following chapters, and appropriate treatments outlined and explained. The vital point to remember when treating an impairment in any one of the particular systems is that once one is affected, the others will begin to show their own symptoms. The initial priority of all first aid is the monitoring and treatment of the three major systems above all else.

However, before any medical assessment can be made, and any particular treatment delivered, the first aider must have a systematic, accurate, and comprehensive method of diagnosis.

DIAGNOSTIC PROCEDURES

Diagnosis is obviously the basis of all subsequent medical treatment, and its accuracy is vital. Making a survival first aid diagnosis, though, is rather different from the diagnosis made by a doctor in a casualty department, who can make judgments with great accuracy and speed. On the top of a mountain far from a hospital, your diagnosis of someone with abdominal pain might be just that – you acknowledge their abdominal pain, check for potentially dangerous conditions such as appendicitis, monitor their other vital signs and then, if there are no further complications, accept that there is little more you can do.

Yet there is still a great deal you can tell about a patient's condition by a careful observation of the physical signs displayed. But take note. Only once you have assessed potential or actual life-threatening conditions, and treated them, should you concern yourself with less life-threatening conditions and what you can do about them. You should think of your diagnostic procedure falling into four distinct types:

- **Emergency assessment** – the most important and always the first! An examination of the patient's vital signs to detect dangerous injuries or illnesses which need immediate treatment.

- **Comprehensive assessment** – a head-to-toe examination of the patient with a view to gaining the fullest possible understanding of his or her medical condition in order to extend the treatment. Before examination, take the patient's history (if conscious).
- **Historical assessment** – gathering background information on the causes behind the injury or illness to guide further treatment.
- **Environmental assessment** – an assessment peculiar to survival first aid. Make a diagnosis of how your environment contributes to your immediate and extended treatment of the patient.

Clearly, these types of assessment are not rigidly separated, and may overlap depending on the circumstances. Be flexible, but always make your emergency assessment first if the accident is serious. If the patient's circulatory, respiratory, or nervous system is failing, every other medical issue is secondary until he or she is stabilized.

EMERGENCY DIAGNOSIS – READING THE VITAL SIGNS

Upon first reaching a casualty, your instant reaction may be one of mental paralysis, especially if the injuries are severe and gruesome, or if the patient is making a great deal of noise on account of his or her pain. Bloody or messy wounds will rightly attract your attention, but on the issue of pain you may have to take a harder attitude. This is especially true if there are multiple casualties. If a casualty is shouting or screaming, then at the very least you know that his or her airway is open, and he or she is conscious and breathing. Your attention should go more towards those who are unconscious and silent – they may well be in more imme-

diate life-threatening danger (though naturally you must not ignore those who are pleading with you for help).

Upon reaching any patient with a substantial injury or illness, the first diagnostic action you must make is to check his Airway, Breathing, and Circulation. These are not the only diagnostic actions you must make in the course of assessing the vital signs, but the ABC abbreviation will help you bring them easily to mind even when you are in a traumatic situation. They also take you straight to the nub of any truly serious problems.

Airway

If a person is unconscious, the loss of muscular control in the tongue means that it can drop back and form a soft, but effective, plug at the entrance to the airway and prohibit respiration. Other objects such as food or false teeth could also be lodged there. One of your first actions then should be to open the casualty's mouth and inspect for any blockages. Clear the mouth of any obvious blood, vomit, or foreign bodies, and ease the tongue forward to open the airway. To keep the airway open, you must slightly reposition the casualty's head. Place one hand on the casualty's forehead, and put two fingers from the other hand under the point of his chin. Gently tilt the head backwards to a shallow angle, moving the head very slowly and carefully in case there are any spinal or neck injuries. This will open the airway enough for the patient to breathe on his or her own. Place the patient in the recovery position to assist a natural breathing action (see box).

It may be that the patient has a more securely lodged obstruction in the throat or deeper down the windpipe. In this case, you may have to use more forcible methods of removal such as the Heimlich manoeuvre or a variant. Consult Chapter Three for full details on how to practice these techniques.

If you are especially well prepared you may be carrying an artificial airway and a

Opening the airway and checking breathing

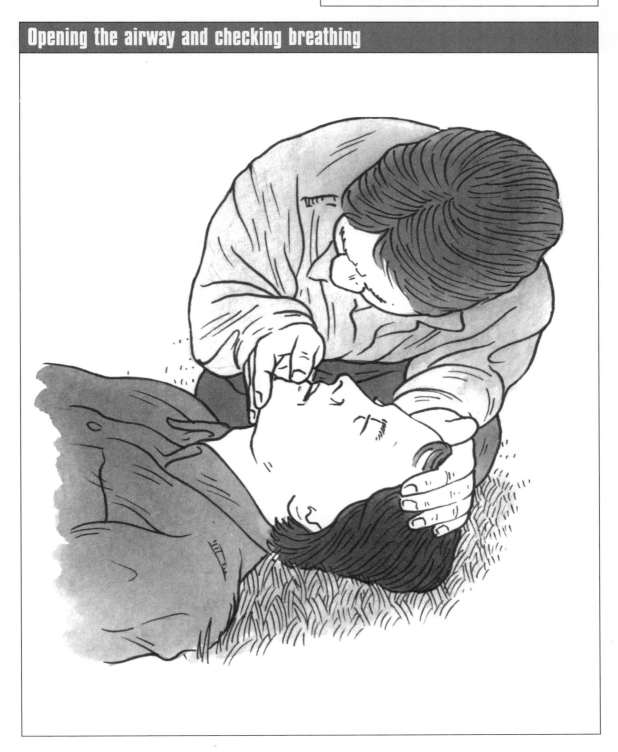

Using a blood pressure cuff

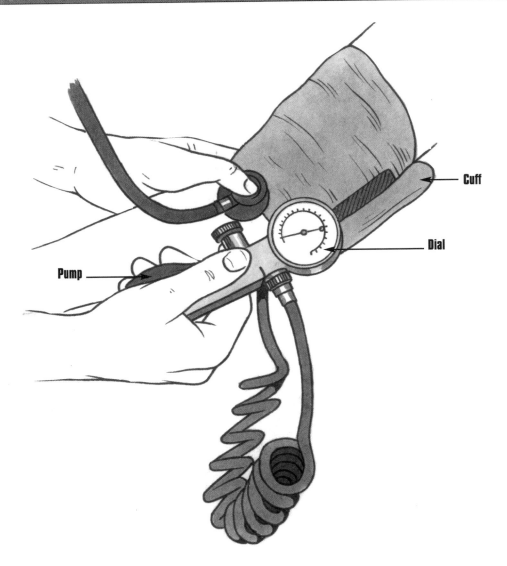

Cuff

Dial

Pump

In an emergency, a systolic blood pressure reading is important and can be gained using a blood pressure cuff. Wrap the cuff around the casualty's upper arm, and pump it tight until arterial blood flow to the arm is stopped (the pulse in the wrist stops). Slowly deflate the cuff while feeling for the return of the pulse (or use a stethoscope to do this). As soon as you feel the pulse return, take a reading from the gauge. Anything below 60 is dangerous – it can be evidence of the onset of shock or severe blood loss.

mucus extractor in your medical pack. The artificial airway is essentially a tube inserted down the patient's windpipe to give a clear breathing passage. Learn how to use it before any real emergency. The basic principle is to place one third of the tube's length into the patient's mouth pointing towards the roof of the mouth, then turn the tube 180 degrees so that the rest of the tube can be smoothly guided down the patient's throat to open up an airway. Once this is in place, a mucus extractor can be used – the one-way extractor enables you to suck out any fluid blockages without fear of contamination.

Breathing

Once the airway has been cleared (remember that this should be done in seconds) check the casualty's breathing. Bend down and place your cheek right next to the casualty's mouth and nose while keeping your eyes on the casualty's chest. This will allow you three opportunities to detect lack of breathing – you should feel the casualty's breath on your cheek, hear it, and also see the rise and fall of the chest, which should be equal on both sides. If all these signs are absent for over 10 seconds, then you can judge the breathing to have stopped and you can start giving resuscitation (see Chapter Three). Remember, though, that you are also looking for respiratory distress as well as respiratory failure. If the breathing is abnormally sluggish, laboured, or weak, then you may have cause to give mouth-to-mouth ventilation as an aid to the casualty's own attempts.

Circulation

The basic principle here is to check for any major sources of blood or fluid loss, and to monitor the heartbeat. Checking for blood loss simply involves finding any source of heavy bleeding and stemming the flow with whatever technique is appropriate (see Chapters Three and Four). This is imperative in stopping physiological shock setting in. In

a survival situation in a cold climate you must be especially diligent in checking all areas of the body, as heavy layered clothing which is waterproof can often keep sites of bleeding well hidden. Checking for the pulse can be done at one of two places. The first is the radial artery in the wrist. Take three fingers (never your thumb, as this has a pulse of its own which may confuse matters) and place them over the artery situated on the inside of the wrist, about 1cm (0.5in) in from the thumb side (if you cross the central tendon you have gone too far). The other, preferable, location for the pulse is the main artery in the neck. This is found simply by running your fingers down the back angle of the jaw and descending onto the neck until your fingers drop into the groove along the side of the throat. There you should feel a pulse. If the casualty is a man, you can also find the pulse by sliding the fingers from the Adam's apple just to the side of the throat. If you can find no pulse for a period of 10 seconds, then you should judge that the heart has stopped and begin resuscitation (see Chapter Three). But even if a pulse is found, monitor it very regularly to check for changes in condition. Practice finding these pulse signatures on yourself and a colleague before you set out.

Also, check for signs of circulation if it is difficult to check properly for a pulse. If such signs are present, resuscitation may not be required.

The ABC assessments may sometimes have to be performed out of sequence, depending upon the condition of the casualty. These three simple checks are life savers in their own right, but for a complete diagnosis of the casualty's vital signs you may have to go further.

Consciousness

The degree of consciousness of a casualty can be assessed fairly accurately using the AVPU scale:

Finding the pulse on wrist or neck

Take three fingers (never your thumb) and place them over the artery situated on the inside of the wrist (A), about 1cm (0.5in) in from the thumb side.

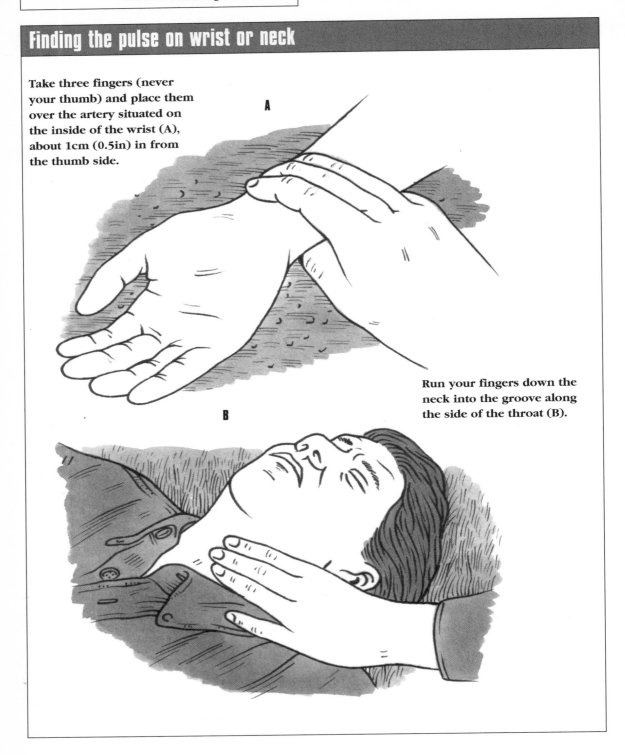

Run your fingers down the neck into the groove along the side of the throat (B).

A = Alert The casualty is fully conscious, aware of his position, and is able to interact fully with the outside world. The diagnostic process for this is simply that you can interact with the person as usual.

V = Voice At this level of consciousness, the casualty is still responding to your voice, though they may be sluggish or incoherent. To test this level of response, give the person simple commands to follow, such as getting them to blink their eyes or squeeze your hand if they can hear you.

P = Pain Here the casualty will only seem to respond to pain. Try inducing particularly sensitive pains or sensations, such as squeezing the ear lobe or scratching the soles of the feet. If the person tries to pull away or they move, then there is still activity being processed between the nerves, spinal cord, and brain.

U = Unresponsive This is a very serious state in which the casualty is totally unconscious, and does not react to any form of stimulus.

The AVPU scale is useful in that it helps you to judge the condition of the nervous system, and to derive information about the casualty's wider injuries or illness.

Temperature

The healthy human body stays in a core temperature range of 36–38°C (97.8–100.4°F). Anything above or below this is a serious risk to the patient's health. Thus having a thermometer in your first aid pack is invaluable, if not essential, because of the greater risk of temperature-related disorders in outdoor survival situations. To use a mercury thermometer, first shake it well, holding it at the opposite end to the silver mercury bulb, until the temperature reading drops below the 36°C (97.8°F) mark. Then place the thermometer, bulb end first, either under the tongue or under the armpit (use the latter if there is a danger of the patient biting, such as

during a convulsion). Leave it there for three minutes, then read it.

Spine

With the all-important spinal column running up the vertebrae, the condition or position of the spine is one of your primary diagnostic checks. The essential principle is that if the casualty has been in an accident which may have implicated the spine, then do not move them unless they are in imminent danger from some other source. Your basic intention should be to keep the spine and neck aligned and protected from any further movement. The procedures for this can be found in Chapter 7, but from a diagnostic point of view, you should take very seriously any pain the casualty reports in the back or neck area, or sensations such as numbness or pins and needles in the limbs, which may indicate a breakdown in nerve-spinal cord transmissions.

The diagnostic techniques outlined above should be sufficient to alert you to the most immediately life-threatening or acute conditions that you might face. For survival purposes, remember that any of the patient's clothing you have removed may need to be replaced, or the injured area covered by some other means. The casualty is still at risk from elements such as sunburn or exposure even though they are already injured.

The diagnosis of vital signs should be repeated every few minutes or as appropriate to the casualty's condition. One diagnostic run will give you a snapshot of the victim's condition at that particular moment, but continual assessments enable you to judge how the casualty's condition is progressing, and allow you to adapt your treatments accordingly. It will also give you more details to give to the rescue services when they arrive. For this reason, consider a pad and a pencil (not a pen, which can fail) as being part of your first aid kit. It will be hard enough to perform the necessary treatments over several hours without having to remember the details of temperature and pulse rate.

Top-to-toe diagnosis

The vital signs procedures outlined above are not the limits of your diagnosis. Once the patient's most immediate needs are attended to, then you should, if appropriate, do a full check of their condition from head to toe looking for the following injuries or disorders:

● **Head** – look for bleeding from the face or scalp; blood or fluid leaking from the nose or ears (can in certain situations indicate an injury to the skull or brain); eyes – check for foreign objects, and also look closely to see if the pupils are significantly different in size (suggestive of brain injury or stroke); test to see whether the casualty can move his or her eyes in regular patterns from side to side and up and down (if not, this could again indicate brain damage); ask the casualty about any problems with vision; examine the condition or shape of the jaw for any breakages or dislocations; assess if the face is symmetrical (if one side of the face droops or is less controlled, a stroke is a likely cause); look for mouth injuries such as lost teeth or heavy gum bleeding.

● **Skin** – firstly examine the skin for any unusual coloration or tint. If the person has dark skin, look at pale parts of the body such as the soles of feet, inside of lips or eyelids, or finger/toe nails. The following colorations may be present:

blue or blue/grey: especially if prominent in the lips and fingernails, can indicate hypoxia, disrupted breathing, heart attack, or other cardiac problems. If the person is unconscious and there are other environmental indications, this may be indicative of cerebral malaria.

darkened skin: can be a symptom of starvation.

pale skin: if combined with cool, moist texture, suggests shock; in the lips or eyelids, can indicate anaemia. Skin lightening can also occur with a lack of nutritional protein; hypothermia.

red: fever; heat-stroke; sunburn.

yellow: diseases of the liver such as hepatitis, cirrhosis, diseases of the gallbladder.

Skin colour is not the only focus of your diagnosis. Look also for swollen lymph

Main areas for diagnosis

Any first aid assessment should follow a methodical process of examination. The immediate priority should be to assess the main vital systems (A) then proceed to examine the entire body surface (B).

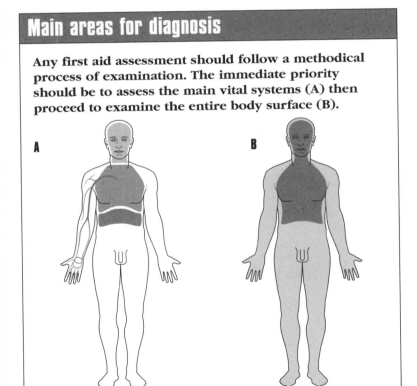

A

B

Removing a helmet while stabilizing the neck

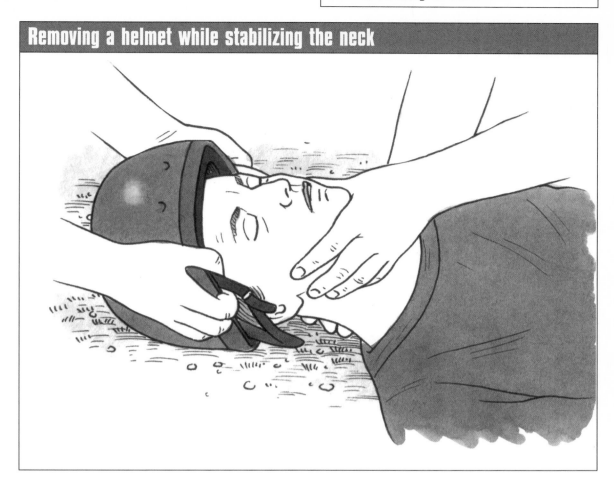

nodes in the neck, armpit, or groin (see illustration for locations), which indicate the fighting of a virus or infection. The particular lymph nodes that are swollen will usually indicate the proximity of the infection. Be aware of rashes, especially if they coincide with any other symptoms of contact with external materials. In tropical parts of the world, look for lumps or bumps which may be caused by parasites.

- **Neck** – do not manipulate, but feel along the top part of the spine for irregularities. Check the windpipe visually for any bruisings, swellings, markings, and so on.
- **Chest** – it is very important to see that both sides of the chest move equally when breathing. Listen to the chest for any wheezings, cracklings, or whistlings which may indicate the presence of fluid. Look for a sucking-in effect between the ribs and at the bottom of the neck behind the collar bone. This usually means that air is not getting through properly. Check visually for any damage.
- **Arms and hands** – Check visually for any breakages or swellings. Examine fingernails for any blueness indicative of a circulatory/respiratory disorder. Ask the casualty about any unusual sensations (numbness, pins and needles) to judge if any nerve or spinal damage. Have the

Lymph-node locations

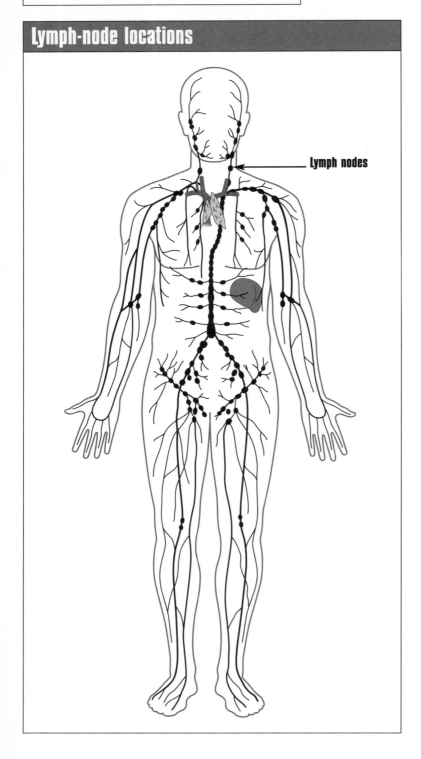

Lymph nodes

casualty squeeze your two forefingers, and note any dissimilarity in grip strength between the two hands (which could indicate a brain impairment such as stroke or physical damage to the limb).

● **Abdomen** – Check for unusual swellings or marks, or if the abdomen is very hard or rigid (could indicate such illnesses as peritonitis). If there is pain, note its location by pressing gently and getting the patient to respond. If the person has not passed a stool for some time, then an obstructed gut could be the cause (though there would usually be other symptoms as well such as severe vomiting).

● **Pelvic/genital area** – Note any bleeding or significant fluid loss from the orifices which could indicate internal injuries or infections. Are any scabs, rashes or marks present that may indicate a sexual disease?

● **Legs and feet** – If the casualty is walking, get them to walk in a straight line to check their balance. If they are conscious and lying down, get them to pull and push their feet backwards and forwards against the resistance of your hands – note any differences

Two-finger grip test

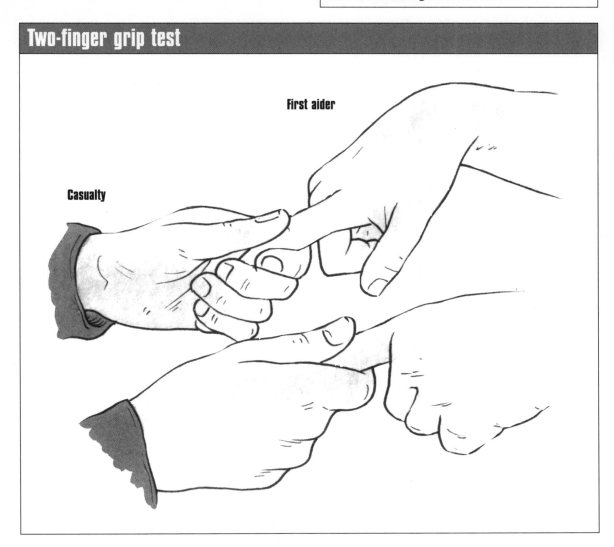

First aider

Casualty

between the strength levels of the two limbs which may indicate nerve/spinal damage. Check nerve responses by scratching the soles of the feet to see the tickle response.

HISTORICAL AND ENVIRONMENTAL DIAGNOSIS

There are two other elements to your effective diagnosis of any casualty that complete the picture of how you will proceed with your treatment.

One, historical assessment, is backward looking while the other, environmental assessment, is future looking.

Historical assessment is the act of gathering all the circumstantial facts which will contribute to your understanding and treatment of the casualty, and is vital to survival first aid practice. Historical assessment has two main sources:

● Eye witness evidence from the casualty or those who saw the accident or development of illness (including yourself);

● Evidence derived from a search of the scene, including the clothing of the casualty.

The evidence of the casualty, yourself and others to a particular accident can give invaluable clues to the type of injuries with which you are dealing, particularly injuries sustained from falls. Finding out how the casualty landed from a fall could suggest how his injuries might be presented. Ask as many questions as you can to reveal particular details which could be useful to you. You should also search the victim's clothes for any information about previous medical conditions (perhaps they may be carrying a diabetic or other card) or if they are carrying medications with them (such as an asthma inhaler or an epi-pen to protect against allergic shock).

Use your common sense to find out as many details about the cause, development, and symptoms of the casualty's illness or injury.

Professional stretchers

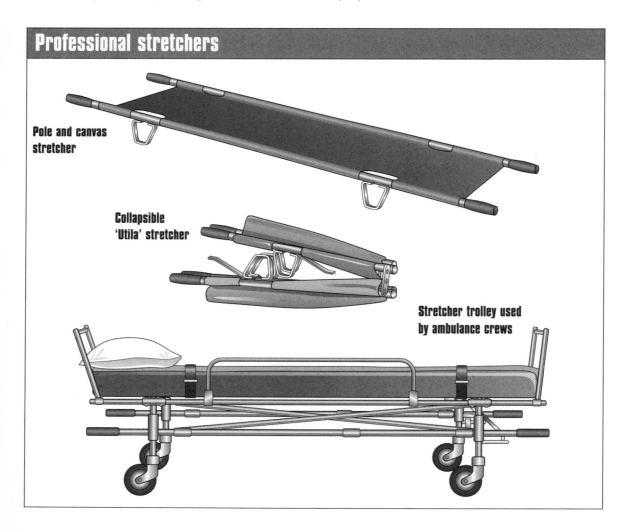

Pole and canvas stretcher

Collapsible 'Utila' stretcher

Stretcher trolley used by ambulance crews

Improvised stretcher

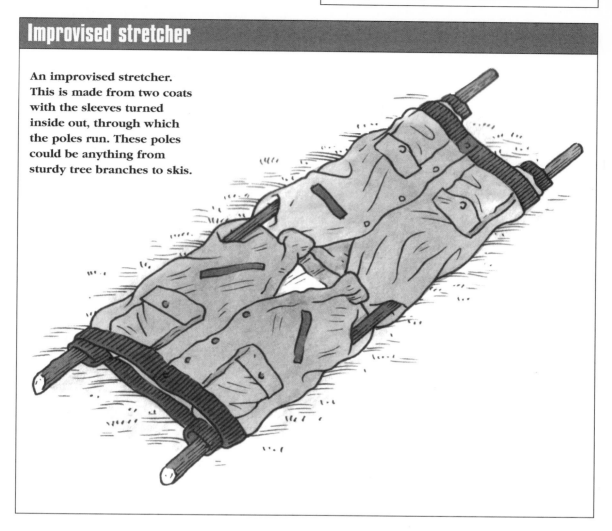

An improvised stretcher. This is made from two coats with the sleeves turned inside out, through which the poles run. These poles could be anything from sturdy tree branches to skis.

Then proceed to make an environmental assessment, though this could be one of the first things you do in the entire emergency proceedings, if the conditions warrant. Environmental assessment is the act of judging the effects of the immediate environment on the casualty's present and future condition.

Typical factors in the equation are air temperature, wind chill factor, wet clothing, effects of the sun, possibilities of animal/human attack (the former can be attracted by blood loss, the latter by your vulnerability), changes in the weather, and the onset of nightfall. Look at how the surroundings may accelerate the problems of your patient. If he is hypothermic or hyperthermic, in both cases he needs shelter. If he is suffering from an anaphylactic shock from an insect sting, make sure that he is no longer in contact with the insect source.

CARRYING METHODS

Moving the injured is a sensitive procedure requiring judgement and, if possible, plenty of helpers. Being in an outdoor survival

One-person lift technique

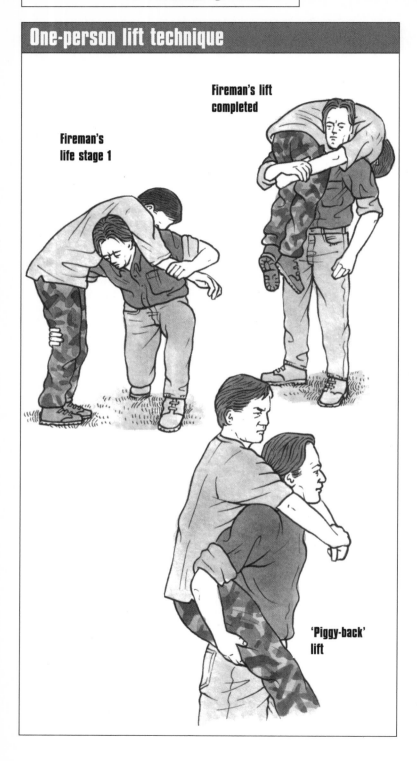

Fireman's lift completed

Fireman's life stage 1

'Piggy-back' lift

situation, the decision to move is likely to be a finely balanced one. If the casualty cannot afford the time lost through your attracting a rescue effort to come to you, then you may have to transport the casualty to safety, especially if you know that climatic conditions will take a turn for the worse. Or your decision to move may simply be that there is continuing danger in the current location.

Your priority is to move an injured person without creating any further disturbance of their injuries. This is particularly the case when the person's back has been injured. Generally such people should not be moved (see Chapter Seven), but if you have to, then split the number of lifters available equally along the body, with one dedicated to keeping the head directly in line with the rest of the body.

Stretchers

If you are going to carry the person, a stretcher is naturally the best mechanism. If you do not have a professional survival stretcher with you, an improvised version can be made using any pieces of strong material (sleeping bags, sacks, jackets) and two improvised poles. If no poles are to hand, roll the edges of the carrying material to create a makeshift handle. Other

Two-person lift technique

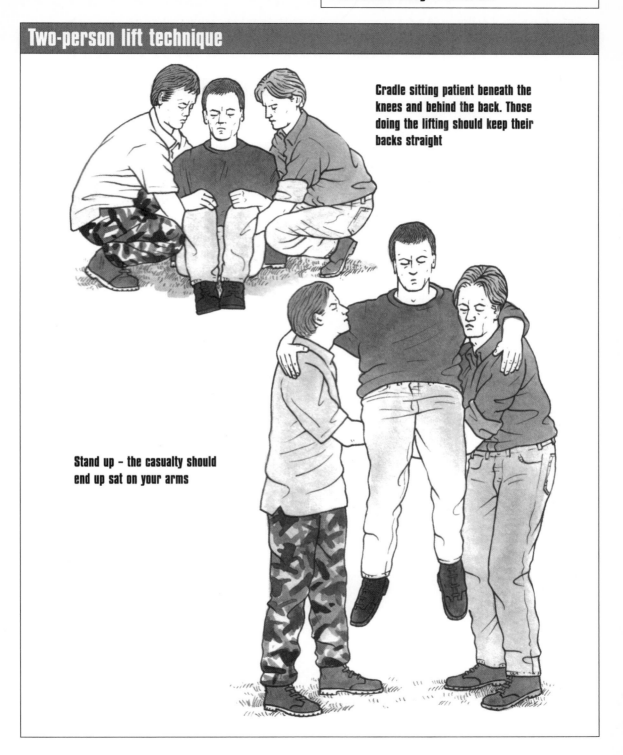

Cradle sitting patient beneath the knees and behind the back. Those doing the lifting should keep their backs straight

Stand up – the casualty should end up sat on your arms

Sheet lift

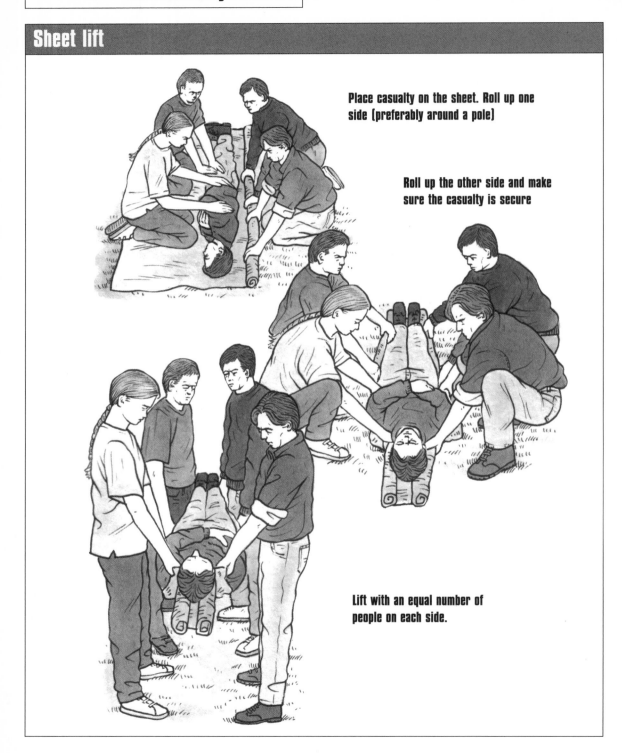

Place casualty on the sheet. Roll up one side (preferably around a pole)

Roll up the other side and make sure the casualty is secure

Lift with an equal number of people on each side.

carrying options include flat hard surfaces such as surfboards, but make sure the casualty is well padded to prevent slippage and motion damage.

If no stretcher is available or possible, you have to carry the casualty by bodily means. This will apply mainly to conscious casualties who do not require stabilization of injuries. However, in a survival situation, any casualty may have to be lifted. Techniques of lifting are illustrated here, but you should feel free to improvise other methods if they become advantageous to you.

KNOWING YOUR LIMITS

Thankfully, most accidents you will come across will not be life-threatening. However, before we move from techniques of diagnosis to the many methods of field treatment, a

note of realism needs to be raised. If you are tending to a very seriously injured person a long distance and time from professional rescue, there is a serious limit to what you can do. First aid can and does save lives, and its judicious application will greatly increase chances of survival.

Occasionally, however, people will die. Techniques such as CPR can sustain life for a significant time, but without the equipment and resources of a hospital, even that will fail to bring a person back to life.

Before moving on to the very positive strategies of first aid, we must take a negative look at how to recognize death when it confronts you. Some illnesses can present an appearance of death even though the person is very much alive deep down. You do not, after all, want to be tormented for the rest of

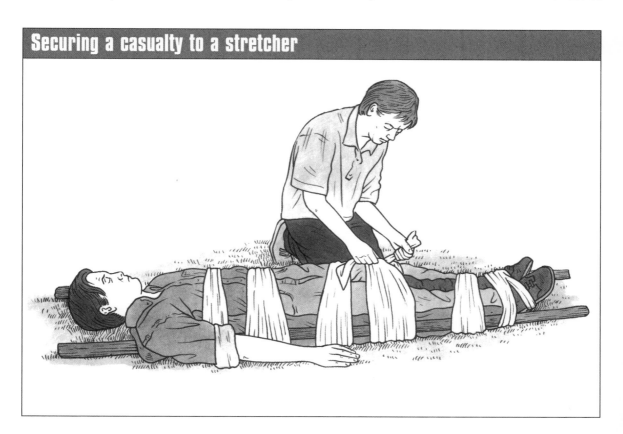

Securing a casualty to a stretcher

Injecting morphine

Morphine is a strong and dangerous pain killer which may be issued to some parties that will be engaged in dangerous and remote activities (it is also carried on aircraft, ships, and by many military units). It is only to be used for treating extreme pain in cases of fractures, burns, amputations, and perforating abdominal injuries. It should never be used on anyone with an injury or illness affecting the respiratory system, as it works to decrease respiration. Nor should anyone with major blood loss or internal injuries receive the drug (children and pregnant women are also excluded).

Morphine is generally injected and comes in pre-filled 10–15mg capsules with the syringe attached. To inject, follow the accompanying instructions and administer to the upper outer quadrant of the buttocks. Then note exactly when it was given and record this somewhere clearly visible on the casualty's person. Morphine will kill in too high a dose, and at least three hours should be left between doses.

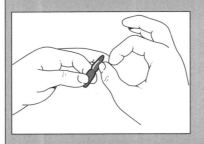 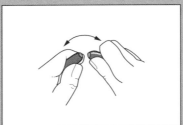 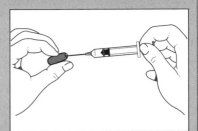

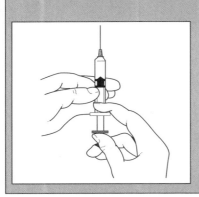 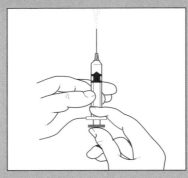 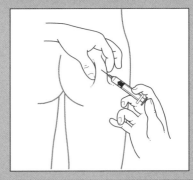

your life about your decision to leave a body on a mountain only to later wonder whether they were dead at all.

Thankfully, there are very clear steps which you can take to recognize the onset of death.

● Cover the person's eyes, then suddenly shine a torch directly into the eyes. If the pupil contracts, there is still brain response. If they remain fixed and dilated, the brain is no longer responding to stimulus, indicating brain death and complete death.

Recovery position

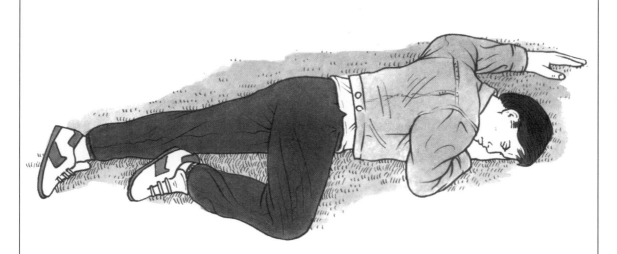

Almost all casualties who are unconscious or semi-conscious should be placed in the recovery position if the type of treatment and injuries allow. The position allows ease of respiration, and also ensures that any fluid build-up drains out of the mouth instead of increasing the risk of choking.

To place in the recovery position, facing, say, to the left, place the person on their front with their left arm and leg bent out to the side at right angles to the body, knee and elbow themselves bent. The other arm should extend outwards, perpendicular to the body. The recovery position

should be avoided if a person has a spinal injury, though support the head in an aligned position throughout the turn (which should be done very slowly by multiple people), and if necessary use padding or your hands to keep the head in the neutral position once rolled over.

● Put your ear against the chest, and listen for a heartbeat (even better, use a stethoscope). Also look along the chest to see if it is rising (do not stare too hard or your traumatized mind is likely to start playing tricks). If both heartbeat and breathing are absent, along with fixed and dilated pupils, death is certain.
● Shake the victim's shoulders or pinching the ear. There will be no response to pain.

Once death has occurred and you are still in a survival situation, try for the moment to

focus entirely your own safety. If you can, note down as much as you can remember about the circumstances of the death as there will usually be a police investigation. Do not try to take the body with you – it will deplete your energy and could become a source of infection – simply mark its location and return with the rescue forces when you are safe.

Having dealt with the issue of death, we can now turn back to the more positive issues of preserving, enhancing, and saving life.

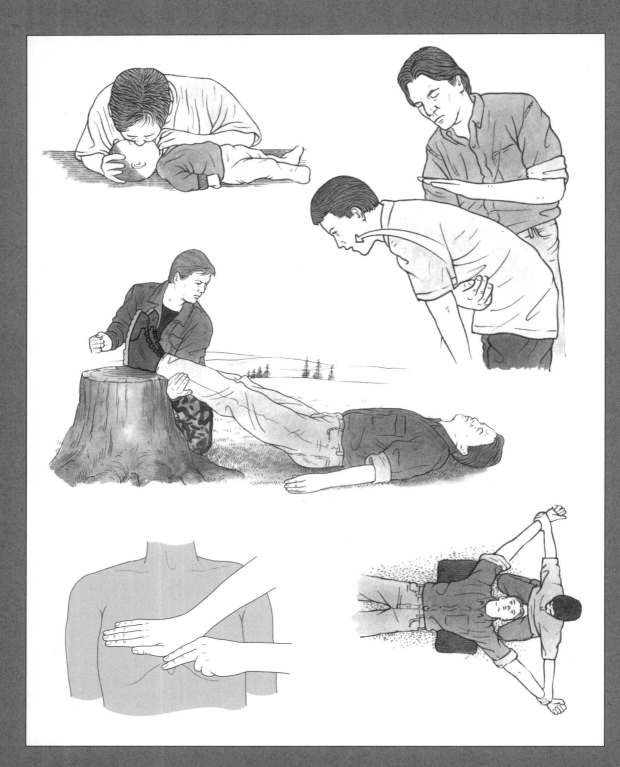

CHAPTER THREE

Breathing & circulation

As Chapter Two has made evident, any problem with either circulation or breathing takes priority in a first aid emergency. Without the respiratory system to take air in and oxygenate the blood, and without the effective circulation of that blood throughout the human body, severe organ failure will ultimately result.

This chapter focuses on the full range of respiratory and circulatory disorders which may be encountered in a survival situation. These range from chronic circulatory/respiratory failures to psychosomatic conditions such as hyperventilation. On the whole, the first aid treatments here are separated into two sections. The first deals with respiratory disorders, and the second deals with problems of circulation. Yet the separation is artificial, and problems with one system will have impact on the other in a short space of time.

CIRCULATORY AND RESPIRATORY FAILURE

Few first aid situations are more serious than the acute failure of the casualty's ability to breath or the pumping of their heart. In this condition, the complete system for blood oxygenation is down, and if left untreated, brain death can occur within five minutes. Myocardial infarction (death of the heart tissue) can follow soon after, and from these situations there is no remedy for the first aider.

Thankfully, such extreme afflictions should be rare if the people in your party are

Silvester method of artificial respiration

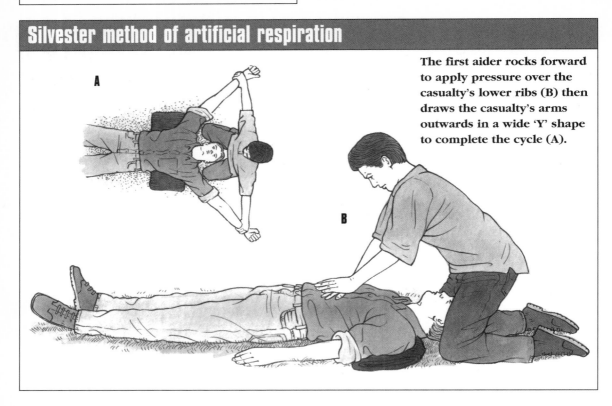

The first aider rocks forward to apply pressure over the casualty's lower ribs (B) then draws the casualty's arms outwards in a wide 'Y' shape to complete the cycle (A).

fit and healthy individuals. The overwhelming cause of circulatory and respiratory failure is a cardiac arrest, or in other words, stoppage of the heart. This can have a variety of causes:

- heart attack;
- major blood loss;
- anaphylactic shock;
- hypothermia;
- tension pneumothorax.

These are the major causes likely to be encountered in a survival situation. Respiratory and circulatory failure at this extreme gives some fairly clear diagnostic signals, primarily the absence of pulse and the absence of breathing, but for the survival first aider there needs to be caution. Especially in cold climates, an injured person's vital signs can become very difficult to

detect as the cold slows down their system. This is in itself an emergency, but make very sure that the person's heart has really stopped before you start pumping away at their chest. If, however, their respiration is weak or erratic rather than fully stopped, the mouth-to-mouth resuscitation procedure outlined here can be used to produce a more regular pattern of breathing.

Detection of respiratory failure
Kneel close to the head of the injured person, and lower your cheek close to their mouth, turning you face in the direction of the chest. Then you can listen intently for any breathing, while your cheek should feel a warm issue of breath (this may be less easy to feel if you are examining the patient in windy outdoor conditions). Simultaneously, watch the chest for the rising and falling pattern of respiration. You can even lay your

hand on the chest to sense movement, as your eyes can play tricks on you. If all these signs are absent for 10 seconds, then you should judge breathing to have stopped and begin some form of artificial respiration.

Artificial respiration

Only 21 per cent of air is oxygen, and only about five per cent of that is used in respiration. The other 16 per cent is expelled when we breath out, and it is this surplus that we use to treat someone who has stopped breathing.

Artificial respiration (AR) is the practice of externally supplying a casualty with enough air to keep their blood oxygenated, and thus prevent widespread tissue infarction. The most common and well-known form of artificial respiration is mouth-to-mouth ventilation. This is when we breath our exhalations into the casualty's lungs and supply the necessary oxygen for survival.

The technique is as follows. First tilt the casualty's head back by placing one hand on the forehead and lifting under the point of the chin with the two forefingers of the other hand. If there are spinal injuries involved, just keep the head in its neutral position, aligned with the navel and the spine. The head tilt lifts the tongue away from the entrance to the windpipe, and allows the free passage of air down to the

Holger Nielson method of artificial respiration

Two seconds of pressure are applied to the back between the shoulder blades (A) then the arms are raised by pulling them under the elbows, but not hard enough to lift the face off the hands (B).

lungs. Then pinch the casualty's nostrils, seal your mouth around his open mouth, and blow. (An alternative is to blow down the nose while keeping the mouth closed.) As you blow the chest should rise – let it reach its natural extent before removing your mouth. Once you remove your mouth, the chest muscles will contract and force the air out of the lungs. Then repeat and keep repeating until spontaneous respiration begins. The pattern you should establish should be six immediate breaths as fast as you can, then set up a rhythm of about 12 cycles per minute. Keep checking the condition of the casualty's respiration using the diagnostic method above.

Cardiac massage

First, the massage location needs to be correctly identified (A), the first aider's body weight should be almost directly over the sternum (B) with the fingers interlocked to provide a cushioning effect (C).

Occasionally mouth-to-mouth ventilation is not an option owing to the nature of the patient's injuries. If this is the situation, then there are two other methods of artificial respiration which may be of use:

Silvester method
Should mouth-to-mouth resuscitation be impossible, usually because facial damage prohibits effective or sanitary contact, the Silvester method offers another route for artificial respiration. Lay the casualty on his back, but place a pad of material under the shoulders to raise the chest a few inches. Kneel astride the patient's head facing the abdomen. Place your outstretched hands over the lower ribs, then rock forward and apply pressure to this area. Then take hold of the casualty's wrists and draw the arms up and out in a large Y shape. Repeat this pattern 12 times per minute, the effect being to use the casualty's own musculature to pump air into his system.

Holger Nielson method
The Holger Nielson method can be used if the casualty must remain in a face-down position (as such it can be a useful technique to use on near-drowning victims), though it should not be used on those with arm, shoulder, or back injuries. Bend the patient's arms so that his face, turned to the side, rests on his hands. Make sure that the airway is clear. Kneel again at the casualty's head

Locating the heart for CPR

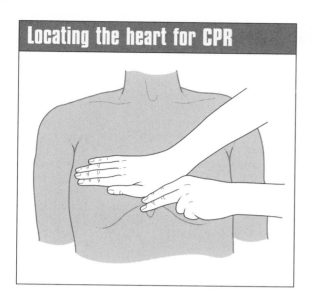

Using a face protector

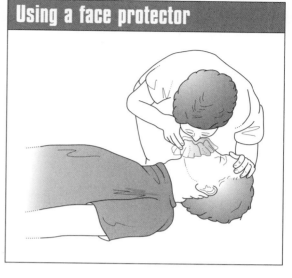

and place your hands over his shoulder blades. Rock forward and apply a steady pressure for two seconds to the back, before releasing the pressure and sliding the hands backwards to hold the casualty under the upper arms. Rock backwards and raise the casualty's arms straight upwards, though not enough to lift the torso or to take the head a long way off the hands. Finally, lower the casualty's arms and resume the starting position. Repeat 12 times per minute.

The Silvester and Holger Nielson methods of AR are not easy to apply or master, and the conventional method of breath introduction is usually to be preferred. Whatever form of resuscitation you use, keep at it. Some casualties have been kept alive for many hours through receiving AR. Yet you also must judge the patient in terms of their overall condition. In a survival situation, you might put yourself and others in intense danger if you stay in one position for a long time, so be honest about your chances of reviving a person. If there is heavy wounding to the chest, and your ventilation produces bubbles of blood, then the lungs may be severely damaged and no amount of resuscitation will work.

Detection of circulatory failure

Check for a pulse on whatever site is available (see Chapter Two), preferably the pulse in the neck. Also look at the skin, nails, and lips – if any of these features become blue, this indicates a lack of circulation. If no pulse is present for over 10 seconds and there are no other signs of circulation, judge that the heart has stopped and begin cardiac massage.

Cardiac massage

Cardiac massage is an externally applied technique for pumping a casualty's blood around his circulatory system in the absence of an effective heartbeat. By compressing the breastbone, which is positioned directly above the heart, blood is squeezed out from the heart. Once the pressure is released, blood flows back in.

Kneel next to the casualty. Run a finger up one of the lowest ribs until it meets the breastbone. Place the heel of your hand about one finger's width above this point, then bring the other hand on top and interlock the fingers.

Lean right over the casualty with the arms straight and press the breastbone down by

CPR variations on a baby and small child

For a baby or small child, chest massage can be done with two fingers or a single hand (A)

and for AR, the first aider's mouth can fit over the casualty's mouth and nose (B).

A

B

A

B

about 4–5cm (1.5–2in). Then release the pressure, but keep your hands ready on the spot, then follow with another compression. Maintain the compressions at a rate of about 100 pushes a minute. This will be exhausting, but keep it up.

Cardio-pulmonary resuscitation

Using both cardiac massage and mouth-to-mouth resuscitation is known as Cardio-Pulmonary Resuscitation (CPR). The interdependence of the respiratory and circulatory systems means that if the heart stops, so does respiration. In this situation, you must delivery two breaths of mouth-to-mouth resuscitation, then 15 applications of cardiac massage, in a constant cycle. Keep this cycle going for as long as necessary.

CPR is an exhausting challenge for one person, and if there is another fit person around, have them deliver one element of the CPR instead of you doing them both. Remember though, even with two people there, you have to alternate between breath and heart massage – the two cannot be done simultaneously.

In all attempts to resuscitate someone using CPR, be honest with yourself. If the cardiac and respiratory stoppage is caused by major wounds, chest trauma, or a significant injury to the brain or spine, then there is little point in continuing. Even if this is not the case, if after 30 minutes spontaneous heartbeat is restored, then you are unlikely to achieve success. Unfortunately, this is much more likely to happen in a survival situation when rescue services are not readily available.

From the acute respiratory and circulatory failure, we will now turn to the other injuries and illnesses which can afflict these two systems in a survival situation.

RESPIRATORY ACCIDENTS
Near-drowning

With the dramatic increase in adventure water sports, drowning is becoming an ever-present danger, even for strong swimmers. Drowning is a phenomenon which takes rapid effect. The sudden shock of falling into cold water can cause a single breath of water to be taken in and, completely deprived of air, the person will lose consciousness in seconds. A further danger, witnessed in about 15 per cent of drownings, is that the throat goes into spasm and closes completely – the person dies of asphyxiation rather than water intake.

Treatment needs to be rapid and decisive. Once the person has been rescued (see Chapter One), carry them from the water with the head lower than the rest of the body to prevent further inhalation, and aid some water drainage from the stomach. Once on the bank, lay the casualty on their back. Do NOT try to pump out water from their lungs using compressions – any water that does emerge is actually from the stomach and compressions can result in the casualty's re-inhalation of these contents. Then check for breathing and pulse in the usual way, but be cautious.

People who have been immersed in cold water have less prominent vital signs, so leave about two minutes for very cold water casualties before judging that heartbeat has stopped. If, however, breathing and pulse are definitely absent, proceed with standard CPR. Once breathing and respiration have been restored, move the person into the recovery position (be careful if the person has tumbled through white water where they may have sustained back injuries), with the head down and to the side to aid drainage.

This is not the end of treatment. Remember that the person is wet and shocked, and susceptible to hypothermia in certain climates. Re-clothe them if possible in dry clothing and place them in a position sheltered from wind. Ironically, the irritation the lungs have received from the ingress of water will make the air passages swell over the next few hours and days, and can produce secondary drowning. So perform your vital signs checks regularly.

Neck constriction

Neck constriction is dangerous because it cuts off the air supply down the windpipe and can also cut off blood supply to the brain by compressing the jugular veins. In the former case, a person can put up a fight for about a minute before becoming unconscious, in the latter unconsciousness will result in seconds. Neck constriction is a particularly prominent danger to climbers, whose ropes may end up hanging, strangling, or throttling them during an accident or fall (also be aware of anything hung around your neck which could catch on a rock or a tree branch). The main sign of a constriction injury is usually something wrapped tightly around the neck, but you may find someone after they have freed themselves from the situation. Other signs of constriction include in various combinations: severe marking and bruising around the neck; unconsciousness; respiratory distress; tiny burst blood vessels on the face and in the eyes; grey-blue skin.

The primary first aid procedure is naturally to alleviate the pressure. If hanging, grip the casualty's legs or waist and lift him upwards to take off the pressure, then remove or cut off the restriction (or ideally get someone else to do that while you keep hold). Be careful once the casualty is released – hanging victims may have a broken neck, especially if they fell into the hanging position, so stabilize the neck as quickly as possible, and do not let them fall heavily to the ground. If the casualty has been throttled or strangled, make sure that the source of their constriction is removed.

Loosen the clothing around the neck and check that the airway is clear. If the person is breathing, lay them on their side in the recovery position. Again be careful in case of neck injury – lay the casualty's head on one of their hands or on a piece of material to stop the head dropping. If breathing is not present, follow the procedure for resuscitation.

Choking and blocked airways

A person suffering from a blocked airway is unable to breath and, unless they are already unconscious, will send out clear diagnostic signals. They will be distressed and red-faced and will usually be violently pointing to or clutching their throat. If they are found unconscious, they will have the grey-blue complexion of cyanosis (the appearance of the skin when suffering from oxygen depletion). Remember that if the person is coughing, no matter how violently, then they are not choking and their body is naturally repelling the blockage.

The most common form of blockage is food, but other causes of choking can be from the tongue, or from a throat swelling caused by an allergic reaction such as anaphylactic shock. For treating a physical blockage by an object, if the person is con-

First aid for choking

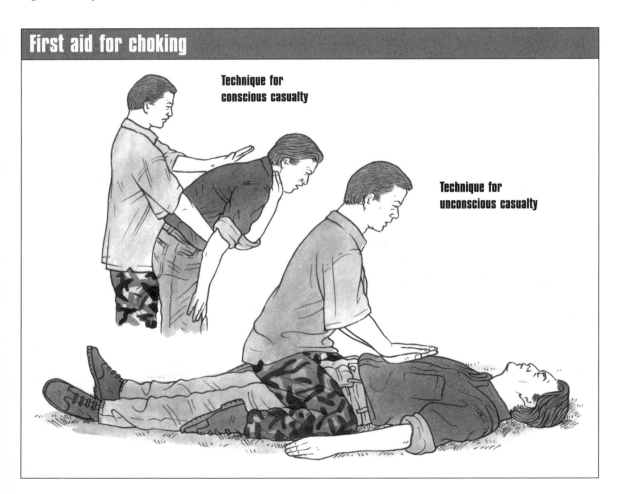

Technique for conscious casualty

Technique for unconscious casualty

scious, encourage them to cough. If this does not clear the blockage, get them to bend forward and give them five sharp slaps between the shoulder blades. Look inside the mouth to see if the obstruction has come forward and can be removed. If not, perform the Heimlich manoeuvre:

Heimlich manoeuvre:

- Stand behind the casualty and wrap your arms around their waist.
- Make a fist and lodge it just beneath the casualty's breastbone with the thumb side against the chest. Grip this fist with your other hand.
- Pull the fist sharply in and up. Repeat three times, then check the mouth.

During the Heimlich manoeuvre, you effectively force residual air in the lungs up the windpipe to push the obstacle out like a cork from a bottle. If it does not work, alternate between the two techniques.

If the casualty is unconscious, not breathing, and on the ground, at first try artificial respiration. If this does not work, roll the person on their side and administer the back slaps to them in this position. If this does not work, roll them onto their back, place your hands on top of one another with the heel of the bottom hand on the breastbone. Now deliver five abdominal thrusts in the same direction as the Heimlich manoeuvre. Repeat this cycle as long as necessary.

Should the blockage be successfully removed, keep a close eye on the casualty for some time, as the throat trauma may cause the throat to swell and respiration to be threatened. Get the patient to suck in cool air to soothe the throat and reduce swelling.

Yet in some circumstances, a blockage in the windpipe just cannot be removed, and a more severe response is required to stop the casualty dying. This involves making an incision in the throat beneath the obstruction, into which a hollow tube is inserted and through which the casualty is able to breathe.

- NOTE: this is a dangerous procedure for the first aider to apply, and should only be attempted if all other methods have been exhausted, and if the casualty is in imminent threat of death.

The Crico-thyroid method of artificial ventilation

Equipment needed: a sharp, small blade – preferably a scalpel or a sharp penknife (not a wide blade); a hollow tube – an empty biro or any form of narrow tubing can be used – try to sterilize them if possible, but do not delay in applying the technique if time is running out. (Do not use unclean vehicle tubes which may impart petrochemical poisoning.)

Procedure:

- With the casualty on their back, tilt the head backwards to expose the throat.
- Run your finger down the throat until it touches the Adam's Apple. Slowly keep moving until you feel another small projection just beneath the Adam's Apple (only a matter of millimetres [a fraction of an inch] is between the two). Locate the small valley between these two projections.
- Mark a depth of about 1–2cm (0.5–0.75in) on the blade with your finger, and then make a small incision to this depth in the valley, cutting into the windpipe.
- Turn the blade sideways to open the cut, then insert the tube at a right angle into the throat to a depth at which it is securely held. This should allow the casualty to breath. Bandage the tube in place.

This procedure is very much a last resort.

Smoke and fumes inhalation

In outdoor survival situations, where there is

usually plenty of fresh air, the dangers of smoke or fumes inhalation are limited. However there are exceptions:

● **Carbon monoxide** – The main sources of carbon monoxide for the outdoor person are vehicle exhausts, fire smoke (especially when burning synthetic materials), and faulty gas or paraffin heaters or cookers used in tents. Carbon monoxide deprives the body's haemoglobin of its ability to transport oxygen. Symptoms of over-exposure can begin with fatigue, confusion, and even aggression, before moving to respiratory failure and unconsciousness. Death can ensure without first-aid intervention. Carbon monoxide has no scent and is very dangerous.

● **Smoke** – any sort of smoke reduces the levels of oxygen in the air and so can asphyxiate. The outdoor adventurer is unlikely to encounter smoke in large quantities, except in disasters such as forest fires or the accidental ignition of smoke flares in confined surroundings.

● **Solvents and fuels** – a major expedition or camping trip is likely to contain several types of solvents or fuels, including gas or propane stoves, glues and lighter fuels. Solvent inhalation is unlikely to poison unless done deliberately, but symptoms include drowsiness, sickness, severe headache, and unconsciousness.

Treatments for any type of dangerous inhalation are generic. Making sure that you are not in danger of being overcome by the gas, fumes or smoke, pull the casualty out into fresh air. If there is little of this available, then at least cover their mouth and nose with a light material. Then follow the standard procedures for checking breathing, consciousness, and circulation. Mouth-to-mouth ventilation could well be required for respiratory distress as well as failure. As in the case of drowning, keep a close check on the casualty for any problematic swelling of the throat, fluid build-up in the lungs, or poisoning.

Chest trauma

Chest trauma can essentially be defined as any injury to or through the external chest wall which impairs the function of the respiratory system. When a chest injury occurs, respiratory problems develop through several sources. Firstly, any significant knock to the chest can create swelling in the lung tissue which in turn produces a build-up of

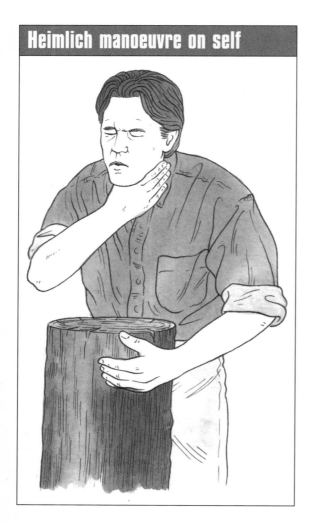

Heimlich manoeuvre on self

fluid in the alveoli. Particular attention should be paid to this when ribs have been broken, or where there has been an especially heavy blow to the sternum. When this has occurred observe the casualty's breathing rate and listen for any crackling or bubbling sounds from the chest. Lie the patient on their side with the injured part in contact with the ground. This may sound unlike common sense, but the ground contact helps stabilize the wound, while gravity also prevents any internal bleeding draining down to the healthy side of the chest.

Another source of respiratory impairment is when there is physically something so heavy across the chest that it stops respiration. When someone's chest is being crushed or constricted, their natural impulse is to breath in to make room – when this is done the weight shifts lower and the person is unable to breath out. The obvious priority is to free the person. If the crushing object is especially heavy, lever it off and prop it up. Then treat any external wounds apparent (see Chapter Four), and attend to the casualty's vital signs.

Two types of trauma

Two major types of chest trauma are the pneumothorax and the haemothorax. The pneumothorax occurs when air enters the chest cavity between the chest wall and the lung. The haemothorax occurs when

blood does the same. Both can occur through external chest trauma, and both have the result of compressing the lung by giving it less room in which to expand, and also to start distorting the alignment of the internal organs, including the heart. In these cases, lie the patient in the same injury-down position as described above. If, however, the chest wall is clearly pierced and the source of air ingress, cover the wound with a patch

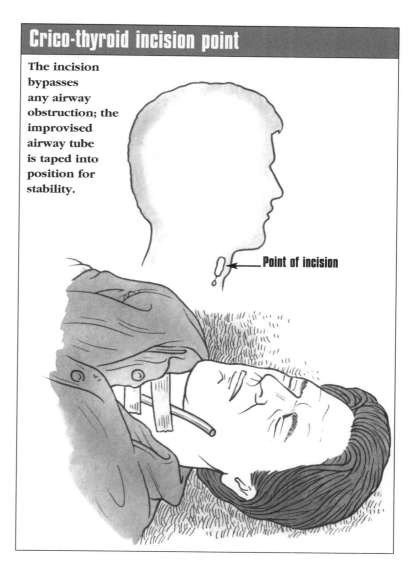

Crico-thyroid incision point

The incision bypasses any airway obstruction; the improvised airway tube is taped into position for stability.

Point of incision

Bandaging a chest wound

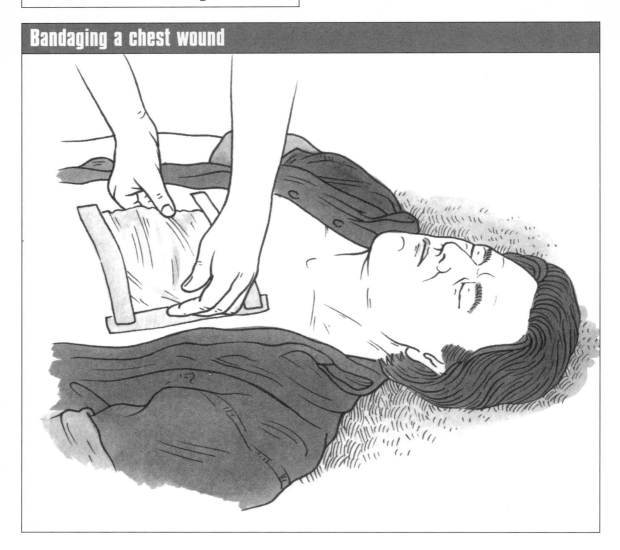

such as a piece of plastic bag to close the air flow. This stops the influx of air, but if you feel that it is making the casualty's condition worse then remove it and simply attend to any bleeding (see Chapter Four for details of how to make this patch).

Respiratory accidents come in several different varieties from those described above, and include those accidents to the nervous system – such as electric shock – which may stop the breathing by implication. Whatever the case, be clear in your own mind about your procedure – make sure they are breathing, if not go to resuscitation. If they are breathing, assist the injuries so that they do not worsen, and evacuate as soon as possible.

RESPIRATORY DISORDERS
Asthma

Asthma occurs with the swelling of the bronchial tubes and the production of mucus by the bronchial glands. Both of these restrict air flow to the alveoli, and so make breathing difficult and distressing, or in some cases impossible. Asthma can be a pervasive background illness, or it can express itself in sudden violent attacks, usually through an allergic response or after over-exertion. The symptoms of these attacks are a wheezy difficulty in breathing and speaking, distress, coughing, grey-blue skin, or even unconsciousness and respiratory failure if the attack is severe.

Most asthmatics aware of their own condition will carry inhalers which deliver drugs designed to dilate the bronchial tubes and aid breathing. Help the casualty to use their inhaler. Also sit them down and get them to take long, slow breaths to calm the anxiety which exacerbates the condition. If the attack does not diminish after 10 minutes, then help the casualty to keep taking their medication every 5–10 minutes while preparing yourself to deliver artificial resuscitation if need be.

Hyperventilation

Hyperventilation is a condition relevant to the survival first aider who has to deal with a panicked group member unable to cope with a dangerous or possibly life-threatening situation. It is an alarming psychosomatic disorder in which a person suffering from severe anxiety or a panic attack involuntarily accelerates their breathing to an unnatural rate. This evacuates too much carbon dioxide from the body, upsetting the chemical balance, and producing symptoms such as dizziness, fainting, muscle cramps, and a

tingling around the face and mouth. There are two levels of treatment. On the psychological side, reassure the person in a soft, but firm voice, preferably in a secluded place away from others. Do not allow yourself to be caught up in the casualty's panic, but tell the person what is happening to them and encourage them to relax. On the physical side of treatment, have the person breath into a paper bag or similar container (beware, of course, of plastic bags because of the danger of suffocation). By re-breathing his spent air, the casualty raises the body's

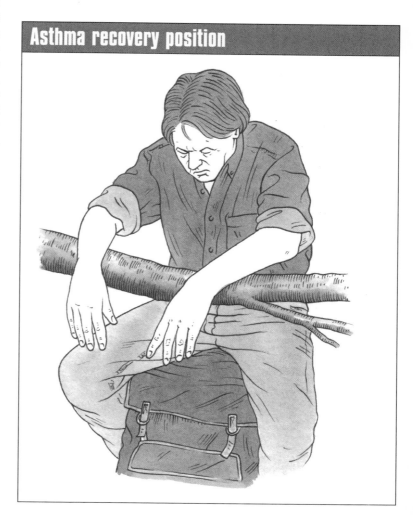

Asthma recovery position

levels of carbon dioxide back to normal. Remember to make thorough checks before classing someone's respiratory disorder as hyperventilation rather than something more serious.

Lung-related illnesses

Though lung illnesses are slightly beyond the province of the general first aider, to the survival first aider they are worth serious consideration. Survival first aid has to include the possibility of long periods without treatment, in an often hostile or insanitary environment. In such a situation, certain illnesses such as bronchitis or pneumonia can develop, particularly if a casualty's chest injury or a severe cough is allowed to develop.

Coughing in itself should be a cause for concern, and at the first signs of its development, cough medication (such as linctus codeine) should be applied if available (it should be part of your general medical kit). However, do not try to stop coughing – rather work to bring up the phlegm being produced in the lungs. Encourage the casualty to drink lots of fluids (or as much as you can spare from your supplies), and if possible breathe in the steam of heated water. Both these procedures should help to loosen chest mucus which can then more easily be coughed up.

Beyond a simple cough are the conditions of bronchitis and pneumonia. Bronchitis is an infection of the bronchi, usually caused by a virus, and it is characterized by a harsh

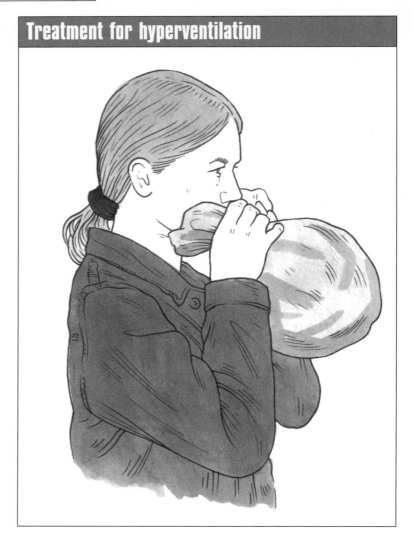

Treatment for hyperventilation

chesty cough and general flu-like symptoms. Bronchitis is a debilitating illness in itself, but it is also serious because it can precipitate the onset of pneumonia. Pneumonia is an acute lung infection and typically follows another respiratory illness, especially in outdoor situations where there is not the rest or environment to recover from less serious chest illnesses. Pneumonia features violent coughing, producing coloured or bloody mucus, chills and fever, chest pain, and a general collapse into intense illness. A pneumo-

Coughing up phlegm

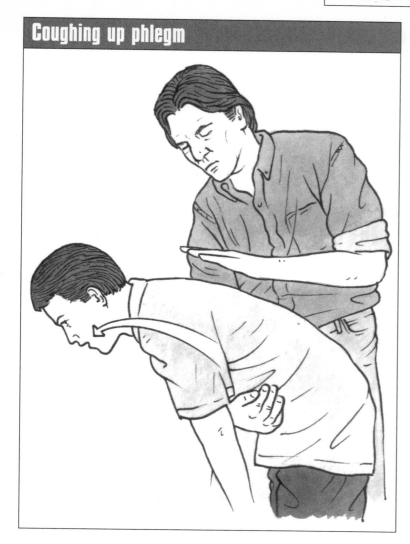

● Get him to lie over a rock or tree stump or other similar object so that his chest and head are hanging down;
● Lightly pound his back, working across the entire surface. This should bring the patient's mucus to a position where it can be coughed up.

With all lung illnesses, if the person is coughing up blood, set your evacuation procedures into action, though you probably would have done so before this stage.

Regularly perform techniques of postural drainage if required, and keep the casualty's fluid intake high. Simple medications such as aspirin can help to keep the casualty's temperature under control.

CIRCULATORY ACCIDENTS
Shock

Circulatory shock, as opposed to psychological shock, is one of the most serious situations a first aider can face. Shock is actu-

nia patient is in a life-threatening situation. Bronchitis can be treated (initially) without antibiotics, but with pneumonia antibiotics are essential, thus as is the casualty's evacuation to professional medical care if pneumonia is diagnosed. Keep the patient's fluid intake high in both cases, and if the lungs are particularly congested, then perform postural drainage. This technique aids respiration:

● Have the patient breathe in hot water vapours to loosen the mucus;

ally the circulatory system's loss of ability to deliver an effective blood supply around the body. This means first that the peripheral limbs and muscles, then the vital organs, suffer from a depletion in oxygen and vital nutrients. This is an acutely serious situation, and can easily lead to the death of the casualty if it goes unchecked.

The causes of circulatory shock are multiple, and can be complex. The major causes for the survival first aider are as follows:

- **Volume shock** – major blood or fluid loss resulting in a dangerous diminution of the circulating blood volume. This can be caused by major bleeding injuries or by severe dehydrating disorders such as acute diarrhoea, vomiting, heat exhaustion, or burns.
- **Anaphylactic shock** – major allergic reaction or a heavy infection can dramatically dilate the body's blood vessels, and prohibit the effective circulation of blood by reducing blood pressure.
- **Cardiogenic shock** – myocardial infarction (heart failure) means that the central pump of the circulatory system is no longer in operation, and so blood is not circulating or regenerating with oxygen.

While the treatments for the wounds and illnesses which produce shock are treated elsewhere, here we will look at the generic treatment for shock. However, needless to say, the cause of the shock needs to be controlled at source – bleeding should be stemmed and any allergic reaction treated.

Diagnosis of shock can be complex. When the blood supply of the human body is first threatened, the body compensates by pumping more blood away from peripheral limbs to the vital organs. Thus the casualty can seem coherent and stable even as they are spiralling into shock. Once shock is established, it can be hard to reverse its destructive progress. So start your examination for shock early, and initially look for the following signs: rapid, weak pulse rate, a grey-blue complexion to the skin in the face, a speeding up of the breathing rate, and a sweaty complexion.

If the shock proceeds, then the person will become weak and less coherent. They will possibly start to vomit, breathing will become weak and speed up, the pulse will start to be less detectable and erratic. At the latter stages of shock, the casualty's mental state will become more agitated and inco-herent, occasionally they will gasp for breath in an attempt to compensate for the lack of oxygenation, and eventually they will lose consciousness. Once this has occurred, the heart will stop soon after.

First aid treatment for shock is possible in its early stages, but once shock is advanced, then professional emergency assistance becomes vital. All the first aider can do is stop shock's progression as much as possible through the following techniques:

- Negate the cause of the shock such as stopping external bleeding or removing the source of an anaphylactic reaction;
- Lay the casualty down with the legs elevated to keep the blood concentrated more in the core organs;
- Keep the casualty warm (but not too warm) – heat loss and hypothermia will accelerate shock (note in step 2 above that you should place something between the casualty and the cold ground);
- Loosen any clothing which may be restricting blood flow around the body.

For mild shock, fluids can be given orally, particularly in the cases of shock where blood loss is not involved. For more serious shock, the casualty needs intravenous fluids.

Keep a close record of all the casualty's vital signs during their suffering from shock, and prepare to deliver CPR. However, at this stage the chances of saving the person without professional help are remote.

CIRCULATORY DISORDERS
Anaphylactic shock

Anaphylactic shock results when the body has a major allergic reaction to a foreign substance. Insect stings, the ingestion of certain food types, or contact with certain drugs are the most common cause of this reaction, but the effect is the same: the blood vessels dilate, causing pooling of blood and lack of circulatory blood volume, while the muscles

Controlling shock through the feet-up position

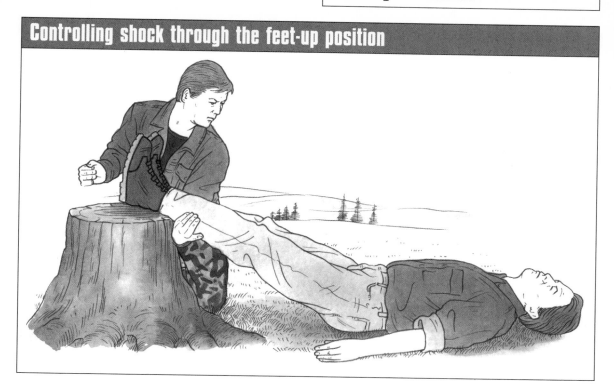

and body tissue swell, often restricting or even closing the airway.

Sometimes anaphylaxis can take some time to develop, but in some other cases it will take effect in seconds. The casualty will become distressed, the face will swell, and red blotches will start to appear on the skin. More seriously, breathing will become disrupted and laboured, and the pulse increases. Unconsciousness can quickly follow.

The best treatment for anaphylaxis follows if the person is aware of their allergy and carries a syringe kit containing epinephrine, a manufactured from of adrenaline. This may well contain instructions for its application, especially with an Epipen which delivers the right dosage. Pharmacy-bought antihistamines can be used as an addition to lesson the effects of anaphylaxis. Indeed, epinephrine can wear off and the anaphylaxis appear again, and using an antihistamine can stop this 'rebound effect' taking place.

If you are in an environment such as the tropics where you may encounter many unfamiliar biting and stinging insects, it is possible that an unknown anaphylactic reaction can occur. General treatments for anaphylaxis are simply placing the casualty in a position in which they can breath easily and, importantly, removing the source of the allergic reaction, such as pulling out the bee sting (see Chapter Nine). Anaphylaxis is an acute reaction, so be diligent in taking away any items of the casualty's clothing which may contain traces of the allergy inducing substance. As always with circulatory and respiratory disorders, be prepared to deliver resuscitation and keep a close eye on the casualty's vital signs.

Fainting and psychological shock
Psychological shock, if it is severe enough, can give the appearance of circulatory shock if you are not sufficiently discriminating in

10 most common causes of death

Although there is little that can be done in the survival context for death caused by disease, the fifth most common cause of death, accidents and external events, can be addressed by first aid.

- Heart disease
- Cancer
- Cerebrovascular diseases
- Pulmonary diseases
- Accidents and external events
- Pneumonia and influenza
- Diabetes mellitus
- Suicide
- Nephritis, nephrotic syndrome, and nephrosis
- Chronic liver disease

your diagnosis. The casualty may seem distracted and anxious, have a pale complexion, and rapid heartbeat. They may faint, the unconsciousness sometimes preceeded by clammy, sweaty skin and the yawning symptoms present in circulatory shock. However, psychological shock is nowhere near as serious as circulatory shock. If the patient seems to be in a shocked condition, carry out a thorough historical and physical examination for signs of injury or illness which could be causing circulatory shock. If there is none present, then treat for psychological cause. This simply involves sitting them down and reassuring them that they are alright, that you are in control, and that their symptoms will soon pass.

Fainting, or syncope, can be an accompanying symptom of a stress reaction, but it can also occur through other routes such as fatigue or lack of food. Fainting is caused by a dip in cerebral blood pressure, and the period of unconsciousness can last up to a several minutes. However, many fainting victims will still be aware of what is being said around them, so talk reassuringly to aid their recovery. The lapse into unconsciousness may or may not be telegraphed by advance signals, such as a complaint of dizziness or a lack of response to your voice. Try to help the casualty recover at this stage by sitting them down, giving them sips of cool drink, and fanning them, but if they do faint lay them down on their back, raise their legs to increase blood flow to their vital organs, and

let them recover naturally. If the fainting fits are persistent, then there may be some underlying serious condition so start the process of evacuation.

One thing to check on a fainting person is the tightness of their clothing around the neck, as this sometimes can restrict the blood flow to the brain and so induce the faint.

Angina pectoris

Angina pectoris is a disease of the heart in which constriction of the coronary arteries means that the individual cannot receive enough oxygen to the heart muscle. It tends to afflict those over middle age, and the casualty will most likely be aware of their condition. If they are, they should have tablets or an inhaler to take in case of an attack, and you should assist in their taking of these when necessary.

Angina is often brought on by exertion, so it is something which the survival first aider should be aware, especially if there are older people in the party. It is characterized by a strong, crushing pain over the centre of the chest and sometimes into the left shoulder and arm. There is exhaustion, a weak pulse, and a difficulty in breathing. For these reasons it can easily be confused with a heart attack, though unlike a heart attack, the symptoms should start to ease after a few minutes. Simply sit the casualty down, get them to relax, and monitor their pulse and respiration. In this way you will be able to check for any more serious problems developing.

Heart attack

We have already explored the first aider's response to a complete stoppage of heartbeat. The most common cause of heart stoppage is the heart attack, or myocardial infarction. A heart attack is the sudden reduction or stoppage of blood flow to a certain section of the heart, owing to constricted or obstructed coronary arteries, usually caused by a blood clot (thrombosis). The casualty will suffer a sudden a crushing pain across the chest which spreads into the jaw and left arm (this can last for up to and over an hour, thus distinguishing it from angina), their skin will start to show the blue-grey coloration of cyanosis, the pulse may become weak, rapid and perhaps irregular, breathing will be difficult and snatched. The casualty may also feel that they are dying and become truly very frightened.

The danger of the casualty's condition is real – as many as 33 per cent of heart attack victims die before they reach hospital. The primary cause of death is a ventricular arrhythmia, either fibrillation or tachycandia, when the heart goes into a rapid, highly erratic and ineffective pattern of beating. Unfortunately, unless you have defibrillation equipment with you and you know how to use it, there is little you can do (defibrillation kits are now much more readily available for public use, and for particularly long expeditions you might consider taking one). What you can do is to place the casualty in a comfortable, stable sitting position with the knees drawn up, and then check on his vital signs continually. Give him any medication he might carry for another heart con-

dition such as angina, and let him chew a normal dose of aspirin (300mg) if you have it available – aspirin thins the blood and aids circulation.

A heart attack can precipitate full heart stoppage at any moment, so be on standby to deliver CPR is the situation arises. After any heart attack or relatively minor disturbance, evacuation becomes a top priority.

As we have seen, respiratory and circulatory injuries and disorders are generally of serious concern, not least in a survival situation where rescue might be a considerable time in arriving. Before setting out of any outdoor pursuit, check diligently amongst your party for any pre-existing heart complaints, and have the courage to stop that person participating if you think that they might be a danger to themselves or others.

Conditions such as angina and heart attack are often brought on by heavy exercise or even contact with harsh weather, and you will need to be stern in restricting participation if need be.

Human blood

The average human being has about six litres (10 pints) of blood. Blood is composed of four different types of cell: red blood cells, platelets, lymphocytes, and phagocytic cells. Red blood cells are the most significant to this chapter, as these contain haemoglobin, the molecule which enables blood to carry oxygen around the body. The lymphocytes and phagocytic cells are types of white blood cell, and these are in effect the blood's guardians, fighting illnesses, infection, inflammation, and the intrusion of foreign particles. Blood acts as an integral part of the immune system. Finally, platelets assist in the process of forming blood clots, and are vital in the stopping of bleeding from wounds and healing. Finally, the blood cells are carried in plasma. This is a fluid which is approximately 90 per cent water and forms 60 per cent of the blood.

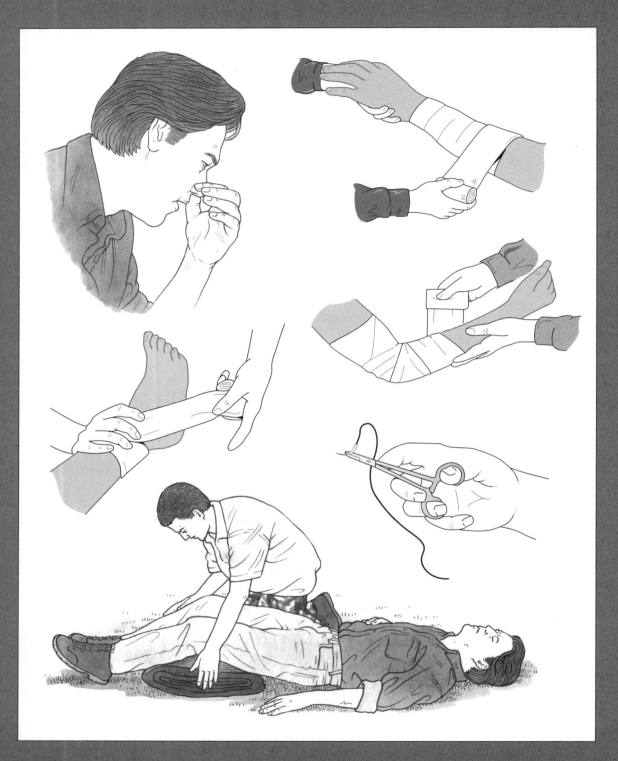

CHAPTER FOUR

Wounds & bleeding

When the body is wounded and bleeding, quick responses from the first aider are needed to stop further damage or prevent potentially life-threatening developments. This means effectively stopping the bleeding and treating the casualty for shock and the dangers of infection.

The types of wound that a first aider might encounter are impossible to summarize, as they range from a minor graze through to major amputation and major blood loss. Yet in essence they fall into six categories:

- **Bruise** – caused by a blow which does not break the skin, but causes internal capillaries to burst, resulting in virulent swelling.
- **Cut** – any incision caused by a sharp edge. This type of wound can have impli-

cations ranging from the trivial to the critical depending on how deep the cut has gone, and what physical structures (muscles, tendons, organs and so on) are involved.

- **Avulsion** – occurs when the skin has been ripped open by multiple incisions or through a generalized crushing.
- **Puncture wound** – penetration of the skin by a hard foreign body that tends to leave a straight wound, of varying depth and damage, into the site.

Types of wound

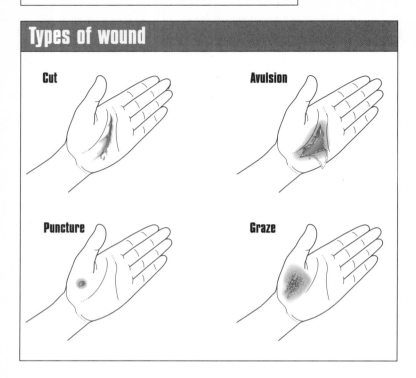

Cut

Avulsion

Puncture

Graze

- **Graze** – a loss of the top layers of skin through an injury caused by abrasion.
- **Gunshot wound** – worth a separate category because of the distinctive type of injuries such a wound can display.

The diversity of wounds means that there are many different procedures for the first aider to learn in order to treat wounds and bleeding, especially as the treatment for any one type varies with the location of the wound. Whatever type of wound encountered, however, there are three main principles governing the treatment:

1) stop the bleeding;
2) treat the symptoms of shock;
3) prevent infection.

This last point is the one most peculiar to survival first aid. Far from available assistance, you may be able to stem immediate bleeding from the casualty, but in the unsanitary conditions of the outdoors you may actually lose them to infections, such as

tetanus, if the wound site is not properly maintained. We will cover the general principles of this in a moment, but first we will look at what happens to the body when it is wounded.

BLEEDING AND HEALING

An average adult human body contains some six litres (10 pints) of blood, which flow through the circulatory system's arteries, veins, and capillaries while being pumped out from the heart. The volume of blood must be constantly maintained at the right level to ensure a healthy blood pressure in the system, and any blood loss through external wounds affects that blood pressure to greater and lesser degrees. The point of danger is reached when the blood loss crosses the 1 litre (2 pints) mark, and volume shock begins (see box on page 82 for effects of blood loss). Stopping volume shock is the primary focus of a first aider when there is major blood loss. Thankfully, however, most human bodies are capable of either stopping, or at least assisting the stoppage of, blood loss.

When damage occurs to any part of the skin and there is consequent blood loss, a clotting process begins at the wound site to help stop the bleeding and form a suitable environment for self-healing. Through a complex sequence of reactions, a distinct group of blood cells called platelets and a blood protein called fibrinogen form a reaction at the site of the wound to create a mesh of fibrin filaments. This mesh, or clot, becomes more substantial as it traps more red blood cells, eventually plugging the wound area and stopping the bleeding (depending on

Controlling blood loss from a limb

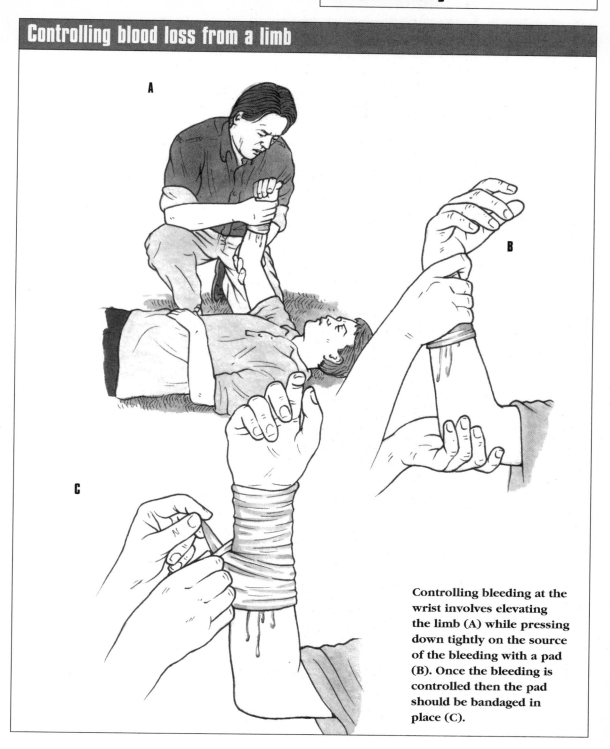

Controlling bleeding at the wrist involves elevating the limb (A) while pressing down tightly on the source of the bleeding with a pad (B). Once the bleeding is controlled then the pad should be bandaged in place (C).

the severity of the injury). The clot serves an invaluable function. In its initial phase it releases antibodies into the wound site, and later, when it has dried into a scab, it seals the wound from the elements to aid its healing.

Once bleeding has stopped, inflammation of the site occurs as a further mechanism of protection. This will continue for some days; as the skin starts to heal, dirt and foreign bodies are pushed out to the surface of the skin for removal, and the wound edges draw together in a scar, and the wound drains of infectious fluid. If no further complications are encountered, the wound will be well on its way to full healing after about a week.

PROBLEM WOUNDS AND GENERAL TREATMENT

Sometimes a wound can be so severe that the body's own means of blood-loss control are overwhelmed. Such wounds tend to be particularly large or deep, or involve a severed vein or artery. Arterial bleeding is characterized by dramatic spurts of bright red oxygenated blood from the wound and are synchronized with the heartbeat. Venous bleeding tends to well out of the wound rather than spurt, and it is a darker red colour because of its deoxygenated state. Both cases are extremely serious as they can precipitate volume shock with great rapidity. Bleeding from these sites must be controlled quickly and efficiently.

The primary treatment for all types of bleeding wound is the application of direct pressure. Lay the casualty down, expose the wound by taking away clothing around the site, and then apply a forceful pressure directly over the bleeding either with your hand or fingers or, preferably, a large sterile dressing pad. Using a pad of material is much more effective than using your own body, and you should use as clean a piece of material as possible to reduce the risk of infection in the casualty. However, if bleeding is

severe, use whatever is at hand – the dangers of severe bleeding outweigh those of infection at that particular moment.

Keep the pressure constant until the bleeding is under control, which should take about 15 minutes. Remember that the success of this procedure depends on accurately placing pressure on the direct source of bleeding, so be diligent in isolating this source by removing hair, washing the site, and so on. If the bleeding is from a limb, elevate it during treatment to lower the local blood pressure and assist your treatment. Indeed, with any severe bleeding injury, raising the limbs (particularly the legs) ensures that the maximum volume of remaining blood is focused into the vital organs where it is needed more. Once the bleeding has stopped, leave the pad of material in place (unless it was an originally dirty material) and bandage it in place. Do not bandage too tightly, as this may restrict circulation which is vital to the wound's effective healing. Once this is done, treat the casualty for shock if necessary, and keep an eye on the bandage to check for further bleeding. If this occurs, place another pad over the top of the existing one and bandage it into place. If you are in a cold climate where there is snow or ice, use a pack of this to further control bleeding. The coldness will encourage constriction of the blood vessels at the site, but be careful not to soak the wound as this will restrict clotting and healing. Slowly give the casualty plenty of fluids to drink after the accident, as the body initially makes up for the loss in blood volume by drawing fluid out of body tissue.

In a few cases where pressure control is not working, a tourniquet is a last-ditch option, as there are severe dangers involved in its use. Because tourniquets cut off blood supply, they can cause tissue damage which subsequently leads to infection and gangrene, and so must be used only to stop immediate bleeding and only if the person is in danger of rapidly bleeding to death. A tourniquet is only applied to the upper arm and upper thigh – nowhere else. It is made by wrapping a piece of cloth or cloth-wrapped wire around the limb several times and tying the loose ends in a knot. Place a stick over the knot and secure it in place by tying a further knot above it. Then begin to twist tighter and tighter until the bleeding stops. Once this is achieved, apply pressure to the wound site in the normal way to aid clotting, and release the pressure of the tourniquet every two or three minutes to stop infarction of the limb tissue. You should be aware that using a tourniquet could cost the casualty a limb, and it should only be used if their life will be lost through any slower method of blood-loss control.

Preventing and treating infection
Most general first aid concentrates on the process of stopping bleeding alone – on the assumption that the casualty will be quickly transferred to the emergency services for professional treatment. The survival first aider cannot depend on this, however, as res-

Controlling bleeding using a pad and bandage

Bleeding from the arm (A) is bandaged with the knot away from the bleeding site (B).

Should blood seep through, another pad (C+D) is bandaged into place (E+F) over the top.

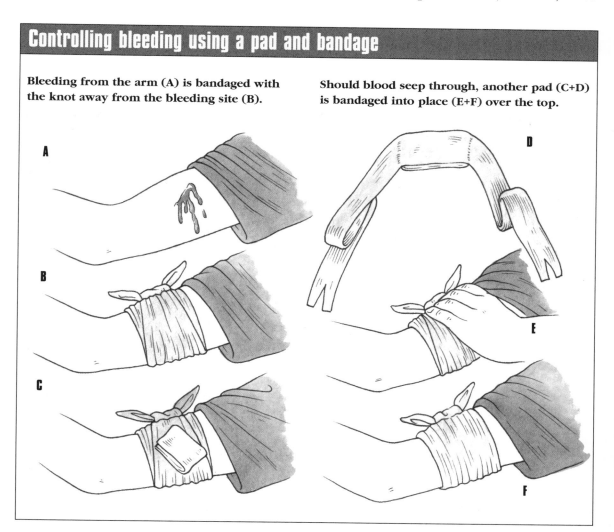

Washing a wound

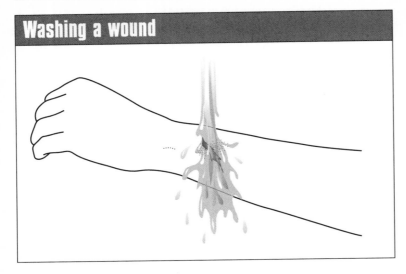

it is sterile; uric acid is mildly aggressive against infections.

You should then spend some time picking out pieces of grit and other debris from the wound. You should have tweezers for the job in your first aid kit, but if not use some other appropriate tool, such as an unused toothbrush. Once you have done this, cover the wound with a new sterile dressing and perform the cleaning ritual daily. With any bandaging, make sure that it is not cutting off circulation – pinch an extremity on the relevant part of the body such as a fingernail, and if the colour does not quickly return then the bandaging may be too tight. In certain circumstances, you may need to close up a wound with stitches or sutures (see box on page 84), but generally the open healing method is best. If you have a course of antibiotics with you and you know how to use them, then do so.

Healing

During the process of healing, all wounds will engender some level of infection. The body's natural defences can handle this to a certain degree, but sometimes infection can become problematic. If serious inflammation and a throbbing pain persist in the wound site over about six days, and the wound is emitting pus and a foul odour, then infection is the likeliest diagnosis. More serious still is if the infection enters the bloodstream and becomes a systemic infection. This is characterized by a deterioration in the casualty's overall health, with fever, swollen lymph nodes and tracts (the latter characterized by red lines of inflammation moving towards the wound), and other symptoms of ill health. Particularly serious is the bacterial

cue and evacuation may be a considerable period of time away. Preventing and controlling infection then becomes a more pressing issue. The overall priorities here are:

● Keep the wound free from the ingress of bacteria and other foreign bodies.
● Keep the wound dry.
● Keep the wound clean.

Most wounds should be washed thoroughly once you are sure that bleeding has permanently stopped. Be careful here – introducing water to a wound may undo the clotting action and start the bleeding again, so wait for the right moment. (In the case of very severe wounds, this might mean that you cannot wash them at all.) Begin by cleaning yourself. Rigorously wash your hands and arms to above your elbow with soap and purified water, let them air dry, and then if possible put on a pair of sterilized gloves (for your own protection as well as the casualty's). Then wash a large area around the wound site. Next, irrigate the wound from a water bottle, wash away the most obvious pieces of dirt, and allow the water to drain away from the site. If no water is available then urine is an alternative, as

Applying a tourniquet

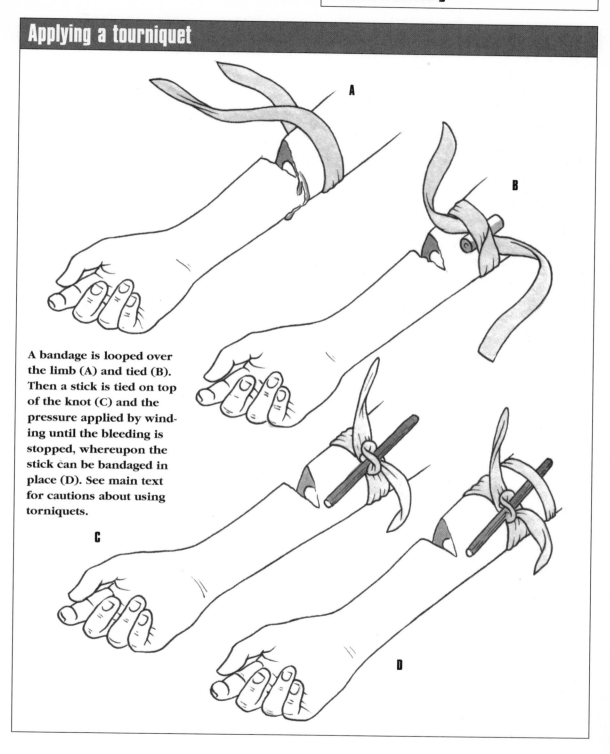

A bandage is looped over the limb (A) and tied (B). Then a stick is tied on top of the knot (C) and the pressure applied by winding until the bleeding is stopped, whereupon the stick can be bandaged in place (D). See main text for cautions about using torniquets.

Applying a roller bandage and testing circulation

Roller bandages are an effective bleeding control tool. Wrap the bandage over the wound (A) before extending broadly to either side (B+C) and secure in place with tape (D).

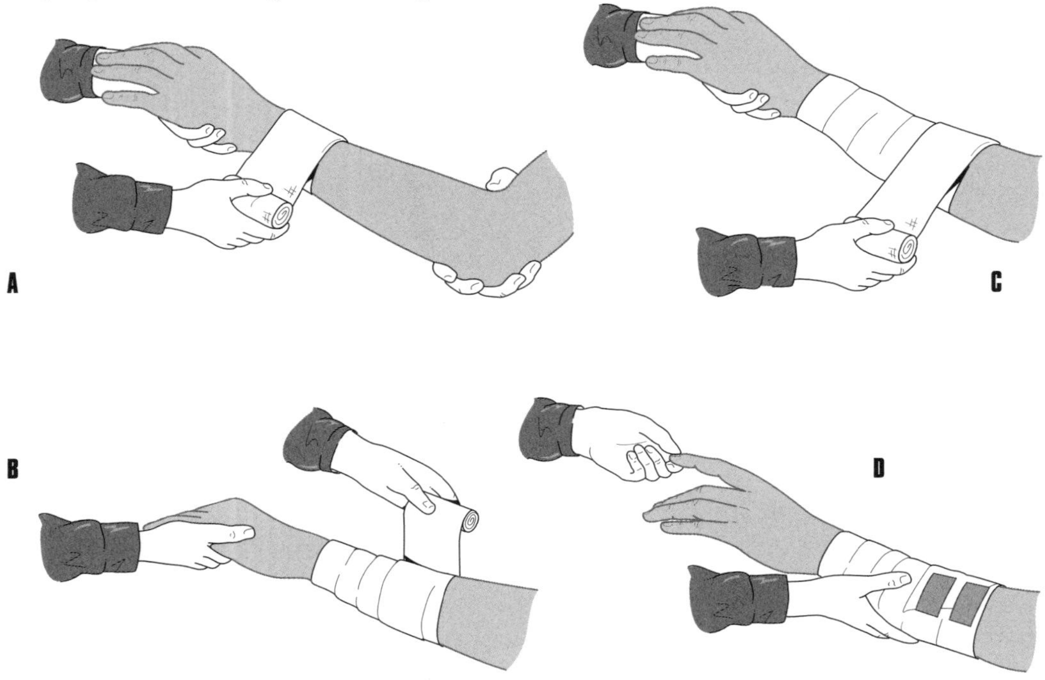

A

B

C

D

infection tetanus bacillus (all expedition members should be vaccinated for this condition in advance). Signs of this are lockjaw and a stiff neck, sudden rigid convulsions throughout the whole body (if the condition is advanced), and problems with mobility.

The types of injury most prone to infection are those caused by dirty sources such as animal bites, cuts that deliver quantities of foreign bodies into the injury, wounds that involve tendon and muscle damage, and ragged wounds which offer the possibility of the build-up of dead tissue. By all means use commercial antiseptics on minor wounds, but never apply them to major wounds as they will result in further tissue damage.

Needless to say, a serious infection requires professional treatment with antibiotics and other drugs. For your part, as a first aider, all you can do is keep the wound very clean and dry, as well as regularly change the dressings. You can also try drawing some of the pus out of the wound by applying a hot poultice. Take any plant or foodstuff that is mashable, boil it, mash it, and while still hot, wrap it in a cloth and apply to the affected area (first making sure that there is no risk of the boiled plant or foodstuff burning your casualty). If no poultice is possible, any heat treatment to the area is beneficial, as it increases blood flow to the area, which in turn helps fight the infection.

Such is the pattern of general treatment and aftercare for bleeding wounds. We will now move on to specific types of wounds and bleeding which may be encountered in the field. The most common types of cuts are, however, the day-to-day nicks and grazes which every outdoors person will experience. The treatment for these is still as we have described above, though the dressing may be a simple plaster. Treat any cut carefully because even a minor cut can attract serious infection. Be especially diligent about this if you are in a tropical climate, where high humidity and abundant insect life make infection rife and healing difficult.

Traumatic amputation

Amputation occurs when all or part of a limb is severed from the body – a traumatic amputation differs in that the limb is been torn off by accident rather than surgically removed. The challenge for the first aider is naturally

extreme. The quantity of blood loss may be less than you expect owing to muscle spasm in the wound area which helps to close arteries and veins. Yet this may not always be the case, and you should go straight into action with pressure techniques and even a tourniquet if necessary. Another useful piece of equipment to have with you is a haemostat. This looks like a pair of scissors with blunt, curved jaws, and is useful for clamping a blood vessel that is spurting blood.

Once the bleeding has stopped, then apply the generic treatment for preventing infection, but be sure that the cleaning process is regular as drainage from the site may be severe. As you may already know, medical skills today are such that limbs can often be sown back on after severing. Protect the limb from any further damage and keep it cool. However, in other conditions where temperatures are higher or rescue will be a long time, do not let the limb

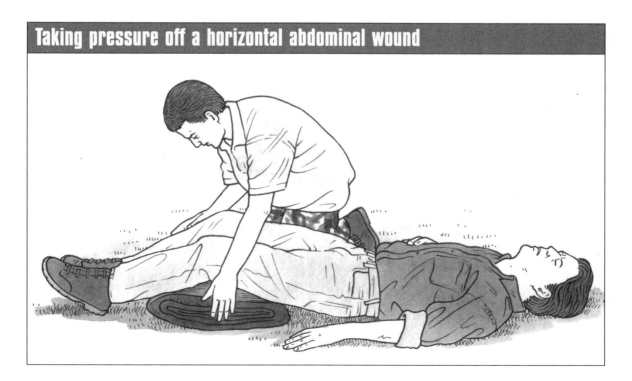

Taking pressure off a horizontal abdominal wound

become a health hazard (in tropical conditions this will only take a few hours).

Head wounds

Any type of wound to the head can bleed dramatically owing to the many blood vessels which run through the skin of the scalp. The treatment is as usual for bleeding, though hair on the scalp can make it difficult to find the source of the wound on occasions, and also for cleaning the wound afterwards. If necessary, carefully trim away sections of hair to reveal the site more clearly, but don't give this priority if the wound is bleeding very heavily; it needs to be stopped first.

Once the bleeding has stopped and the wound cleaned, place a sterile dressing directly over the site of the wound, and wrap a roller bandage over the pad and around the head several times to keep it in place. If the wound is on top of the head, take a large triangular bandage and lay it across the forehead with the loose ends over the shoulders (rather like a loose head dress). Then cross the loose ends and bring them up to the front on the forehead, where the ends can be pinned or tied.

With any bandage, do not bind so tightly that it cuts off circulation to the scalp. Once this has been done, let the casualty lie down but keep the head and shoulders at a slightly

Bandaging a hand

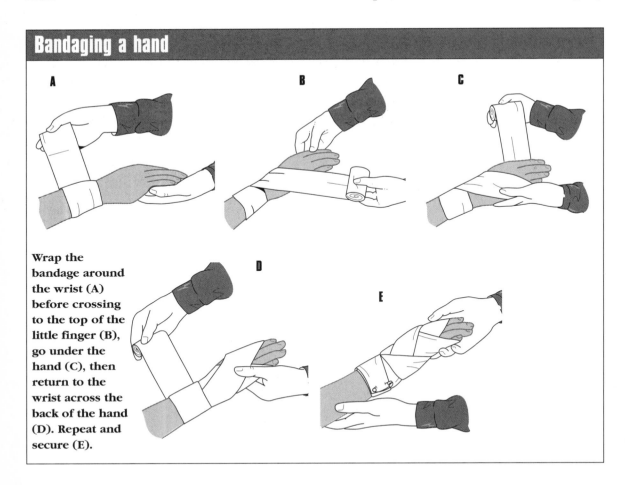

A

B

C

D

E

Wrap the bandage around the wrist (A) before crossing to the top of the little finger (B), go under the hand (C), then return to the wrist across the back of the hand (D). Repeat and secure (E).

higher level than the rest of the body.

For specific treatments relating to skull fractures and other serious head injuries, see Chapter Five.

Abdominal wounds

Abdominal wounds need careful treatment as there is often the implication of damage to internal organs, and the blood loss can be very severe. Sometimes internal organs may actually be visible and protrude through the wound itself. As digestive organs may also be involved, there is a subsequently higher risk of internal contamination, so be on the lookout for any systemic infection if your position will not allow for quick rescue. Pain levels in the casualty may be very high, so you will have to reassure the casualty with a firm and controlling voice.

Firstly, put the casualty in a lying position. If the wound runs vertically up the abdomen, keep the casualty's legs level, but if it runs horizontally raise the knees slightly and support with a rolled up coat or pack – this takes some tension off the wound site. Loosen tight clothing around the waist and thighs, and then start pressure on the wound with a large dressing, using the pressure to keep any abdominal contents in place, particularly if the casualty is coughing. If some organs, usually intestine, are protruding, do not attempt to force them back, but cover them with a dressing and keep the dressing damp to stop the intestine from drying out. A plastic bag can actually be better for this pur-

Bandaging a foot

The bandage is taken from the ankle (A) up to the middle of the foot (B), before being looped back to the ankle (C). Repeat (D).

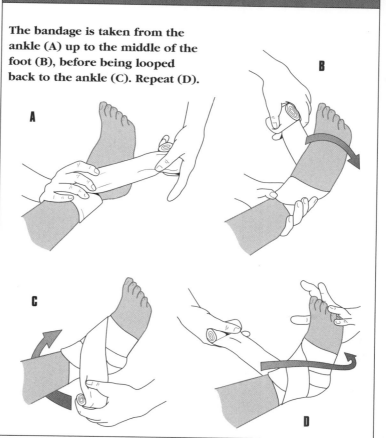

pose than a dressing, as it can prevent drying out without the introduction of water.

When bleeding has been stopped, put a clean pad on the wound and then bandage or tape this in place. Then treat the casualty for shock and monitor the vital signs regularly.

Chest wounds

Chest wounds in which only the uppermost layers of the skin are damaged are treated no differently from any other bleeding wound. However, wounds which actually penetrate into the chest cavity are critically dangerous. This is not only because of direct damage to

Palm bandage

Get the casualty to grip a pad (A) and then bind the fingers in place with a roller bandage, leaving the thumb free (B).

A

B

Effects of blood loss

● *0.5 litre (1 pint)* If a person loses 0.5 litre (1 pint) of blood, the effects are not severe, perhaps just an inconsequential faintness that soon passes (assuming that the cause of the injury has not affected other vital functions).

● *1 litre (2 pints)* Beyond 1 litre (2 pints), the body starts to respond to a more serious challenge. 1 litre (2 pints) of blood loss starts the early stages of volume shock, when the casualty begins to loose the blood pressure necessary for the effective transfer of oxygen into the body tissue. They may become very faint, pale, and unstable on their feet.

● *2 litres (4 pints)* With this much blood loss the casualty can collapse, their vital signs showing a rapid, weak pulse as adrenaline levels rise in response to the danger. The skin will also become clammy and pale as blood is diverted to major organs. The casualty may feel very sick and thirsty.

● *3 litres (6 pints)* With this much blood loss, the situation becomes life-threatening. The respiration and pulse signals will both be extremely poor at this point, and the casualty will probably be unconscious. After this, cardiac arrest and respiratory failure can soon follow.

major organs in the chest such as the heart and lungs, but also because if the chest cavity is punctured, two life-threatening conditions can result: haemothorax and pneumothorax. As their prefixes suggest, these are serious conditions in which blood or air gathers between the lung and the chest wall, and exerts pressure on the lungs, thus causing effective respiration to stop.

Pneumothorax can actually occur in two forms, one (open) where air is sucked into the chest through the wound itself as the casualty breathes, and the other (closed) where air is leaking from a punctured lung into the chest cavity.

Bandaging an elbow joint injury

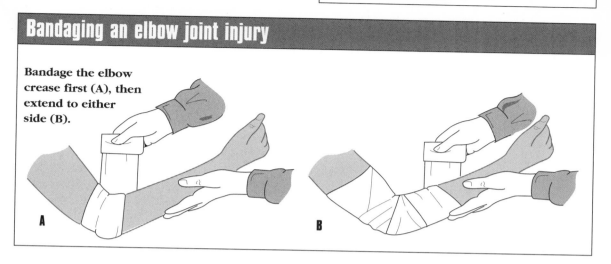

Bandage the elbow crease first (A), then extend to either side (B).

A

B

Both conditions can cause the collapse of a lung, or both lungs if the pressure builds up enough.

Their symptoms include:

- Blood being coughed up.
- The symptoms of circulatory shock.
- The passage of air into the chest wound, causing bubbles of blood and a crackly, aerated feeling to the skin around the wound.
- Respiratory distress.
- Panic.

Immediately cover the wound with your hand to stop the ingress of air. Then cover the wound with a sterile dressing or other suitable material, and cover this with a piece of plastic or other air tight material. Tape this into place along three sides only to give an opening for air to escape with the casualty's expirations – though if the improvised valve seems infective, then tape it on every side. Then place the casualty in a comfortable position with the head and shoulders supported and lean the patient towards his injured side. If the casualty is unconscious, place the recovery position with injured side lowermost, though be careful if there are many broken ribs involved. In both cases,

these positions keep blood drained away from the healthy lung to aid breathing. Be prepared to resuscitate if necessary.

LIMB INJURIES

The limbs are treated very much the same as any other site of injury, except that elevating the injured limb will help to control the blood loss by reducing localized blood pressure as it fights to climb against gravity. If the wound being treated is in conjunction with a broken bone, then splinting the limb (see Chapter Seven) will stop bone movement increasing damage in the wound site.

Wounds to hands and feet

Wounds to the hands and feet are some of the most awkward injuries, as even non-serious injuries can impair the individual's mobility and hamper their subsequent progress, especially if they are climbers or walkers. Also tendons and ligaments may be injured, this resulting in total loss of the use of the hand or foot until professional medical surgery can help the situation.

When dealing with the hands, palm injuries are problematic because they bleed intensely. An immediate measure is to place a pad over the wound, and get the casualty to hold this firmly in place with his clenched

Stitching a wound

Stitching a wound is not recommended for the untrained, but in certain circumstances (and if you have the right kit) it can be warranted. This is mainly if the wound is a clean straight cut which does not go too deep, and is in danger of infection through climatic influences. Do not close up a wound which is dirty or over 12 hours old.

Adhesive sutures are probably the easiest way to draw a wound together. Butterfly sutures (see illustration) can be bought, or they can be made by cutting regular adhesive plasters to the corresponding shape. To use these, simply draw the edges of the wound together and stick across; try to get the edges of the wound as close as possible.

Stitching requires much more skill to apply, and also needs some confidence. Take a sterilized needle or thread (or sterilize both by boiling for 20 minutes), and make a stitch at the mid point of the wound, drawing the edges of the wound together. Then cut the thread and tie it, before making other individual stitches out from the centre until the wound is fully closed.

Leave the stitches in place for five to 14 days (for the face, 5 days; for the body, 10 days; and for the hand or foot, 14 days) before snipping and gently drawing out.

However, before that time, if any serious infection appears you should remove some or all of the stitches to allow drainage.

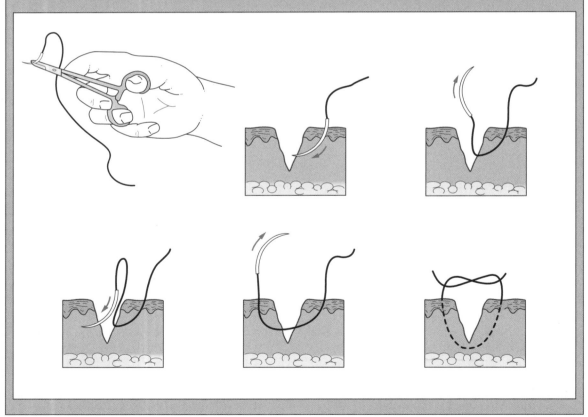

fingers. You can then take a roller bandage around the whole hand including the clenched fingers to keep the tension in place. If the casualty cannot bend their fingers, then bandage the pad in place using a roller bandage. To bandage a hand, start at the wrist with two turns, then go diagonally across the back of the hand to the top of the little finger, underneath the hand and then back to the wrist across the top of the hand in an opposite diagonal from previously. Keep repeating this movement until the bandaging is secure, and pin it at the wrist. A foot bandage follows almost identical lines but starts at the ankle. As with all bandaging techniques, make sure that both of these are practised before an injury actually occurs.

Wounds in elbow or knee creases

Wounds in the joint creases are tricky, both because of their location and also because the large blood vessels in the area can make the bleeding severe. Place a pad in the crook of the elbow or the knee and bend the limb so that the pad is held in place. Also raise the limb according to usual practice.

If the limb cannot be bent for any reason, then apply the pressure yourself; when the bleeding has stopped, put a bandage in place. This should be a roller bandage wrapped from inside the elbow joint (or knee joint) repeatedly around the arm (or leg), working outwards in a figure-of-eight movement to secure the joint and

Gunshot wound profile

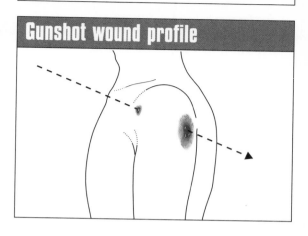

Different stitches

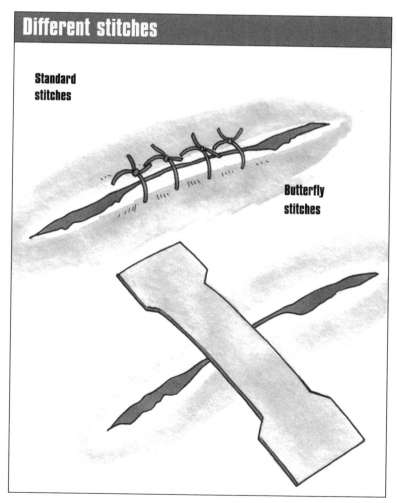

Standard stitches

Butterfly stitches

Controlling a nose bleed

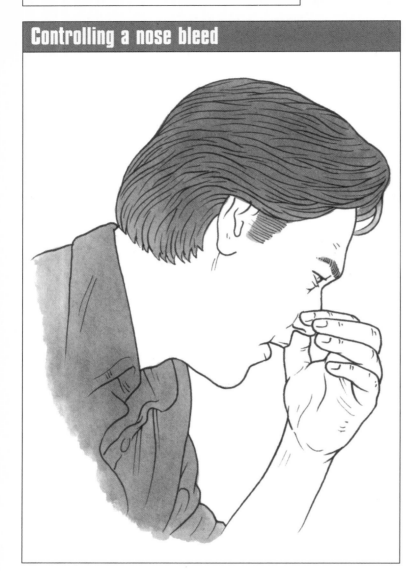

body. It can, however, result from other non-violent causes such as internal infections or stomach ulcers. Internal bleeding is indicated either by bleeding from the orifices or the fact that the casualty is starting to suffer from shock without there being the presence of significant external bleeding. Symptoms can include:

● A weak, rapid pulse combined with a sweaty, pale, and clammy complexion.
● Anxiety and changes in mental state or coherence.
● Collapse and unconsciousness.
● Blood passed from anus with faeces, either as a separate emission or absorbed into the faeces to produce a black, tarry stool. Both symptoms usually indicate bleeding from the bowel.
● Blood passed in the urine, indicating probable bleeding from the kidneys or bladder.
● Blood coughed up or vomited. If coughed up in a red, frothy mixture, it usually means bleeding from lungs. If vomited, the bleeding is usually from the stomach. The appearance of the blood in the vomit can be either fresh and red or like dark-brown coffee grounds, depending upon how long it has been in the stomach.
● Bleeding from the vagina, unless accounted for by menstruation, could indicate a miscarriage if pregnant, or damage to the womb or vagina caused by an infection or other illness.

reduce its mobility. It is very important to check the toe and fingernails to see if the bandage is too tight and is restricting circulation.

INTERNAL BLEEDING

Internal bleeding is usually as serious as it sounds. Most often it results from penetration wounds such as gunshot wounds, or broken bones or other violent blows to the

There is effectively nothing you can do (except summon help quickly) to treat the source of internal bleeding, and the best that you can generally do is to monitor the casualty's condition and deliver life support as necessary. Keep the patient lying down with legs elevated, and keep them warm but do not make them overheat. Check the vital signs every 10 minutes, and put into the recovery position if unconscious.

BLEEDING FROM THE EAR, NOSE, AND MOUTH
Nose bleeds

A simple and common cause of blood loss which can be caused by even the mildest knock. Have the patient sit with their head slightly forward, and get them to pinch their nostrils while breathing through the mouth. Discourage any sniffing as this can allow blood to be swallowed and induce vomiting. Once bleeding is stopped, encourage the patient not to touch or rub their nose for several hours as this may restart the bleeding. If the bleeding persists for more than 30 minutes, consider evacuation.

Bleeding from the ear

Bleeding from the ear should be taken very seriously as it can be a symptom of brain damage. This will be indicated by a leakage of a thin, watery diluted blood – the fluid is cerebrospinal fluid. Other causes include a burst eardrum or a foreign body stuck inside the ear, and this blood will have a more regular texture and colour.

For directions about removing foreign bodies from ears and from other parts of the human body, see Chapter Nine. For all other treatment of ear bleeding, simply seat (or place in the recovery position if unconscious) the casualty with the bleeding ear angled downwards to allow drainage. Cover the ear with a light sterile dressing and bandage or hold in place. Then start evacuation procedures.

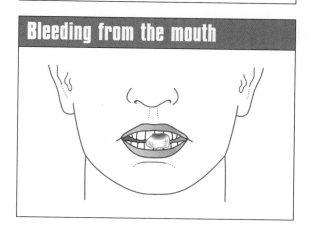

Bleeding from the mouth

Bleeding from the mouth

Bleeding from the mouth is usually caused by either a direct impact to the mouth which bursts a lip, knocks out a tooth or damages the gums, or by the teeth clamping onto the lip, gum, or tongue through an impact to the jaw. Either way the bleeding can reach significant levels.

If the injury is to the lip, pinch the wound between a pad and your finger (or get the casualty to do this for themselves). About 10 minutes of this pressure should stop the bleeding. Do not attempt to rinse the mouth out with water as this may restart the bleeding.

When teeth are knocked out, try to find the tooth and actually replace it in the socket if possible. First stop the bleeding by plugging the socket hole with a gauze pad which the casualty keeps in place by biting on it. When the bleeding is stopped, and if you can find it in an appropriate condition, replace the tooth in the socket and start to evacuate. If the tooth will not go back in, keep it moistened by water, milk or saliva (the latter by placing it in the casualty's cheek), and this may be reclaimed by the dentist later.

When treating any mouth injury, tell the casualty to spit or dribble out any blood. Swallowing blood can induce vomiting, or in the case of severe bleeding, interfere with breathing.

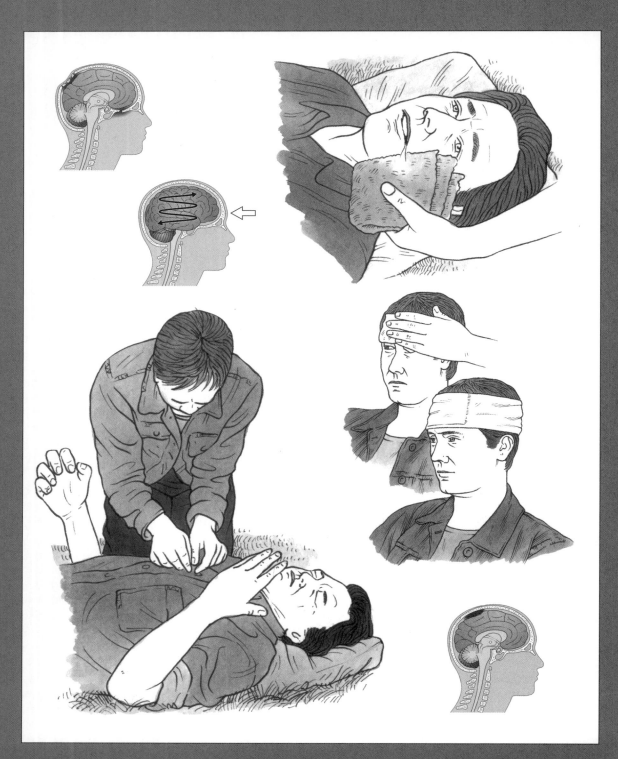

CHAPTER FIVE

Consciousness & head injuries

Changes in consciousness, personality, or behaviour can be some of your first indicators that a medical problem is developing or that a life is in danger. The nervous system controls many of the body's vital functions, from the act of thought to the activities of respiration and heartbeat.

As we saw in Chapter Two, the nervous system in a human being is one of the most complex biological entities. For the first aider, this also creates problems of consciousness some of the most difficult to treat. Essentially, a problem in the state of a casualty's consciousness can occur in two ways. The first way is as the secondary result of some other accident or illness. Thus a heart attack or asphyxiation can result in a dramatic decrease in the casualty's level of consciousness (although there is nothing

wrong with the casualty's nervous system per se). The second way is through a disorder or accident that directly involves the nervous system's function and components. In this category, you will find events such as epilepsy, injury to the spinal cord, and brain damage.

What makes this situation doubly complex is that the two types of nervous system disorder can feed off each other in an emergency situation. So a heart attack restricts blood flow and respiration; these in turn cut off oxygenated blood to the brain, which starts a process of infarction, or the death of the tissue. As this process advances, the impairment to the brain subsequently affects the possibility of restoring normal respiration and heartbeat. And so the vicious circle continues. The first aider will never be able to work directly on the nervous system as they would, say, a wounded limb. What he or she can do, however, is to support the restoration of normal nervous processes by treating the causes of impairment or preventing a worsening of the condition.

We will now look at treatments for most of the major consciousness problems that a survival first aider is likely to encounter.

DIAGNOSING CONSCIOUSNESS

When attempting to diagnose a casualty's level of consciousness, a degree of subtlety is required on the part of the first aider, particularly in a survival context. Judging mental state is not just a simple matter of assessing whether or not he or she is conscious, semiconscious, or unconscious, but also means assessing mood swings, temperament, intellectual performance, energy levels, and social relations. These fine levels of assessment are not so vital to the urban first aider (unless dealing with something such as alcohol abuse), but they are imperative to the survival first aider. Noticeable alterations in mental state may be due to personality, but they can also signal the early stages of serious environmental illnesses such as hypothermia, heatstroke, exhaustion, dehydration, impending convulsion, or altitude sickness. If you notice a change in personality in one of your companions, ask yourself the following questions:

● Has the person been exposed to a particular climatic condition for an extended period?
● Is the change in mental state truly uncharacteristic of his or her behaviour?

● Does the person appear to be confused and less responsive?
● Is their physical movement uncoordinated or clumsy?
● Does he or she appear over-emotional or aggressive?
● Has the person recently complained of, or sustained, any injuries or illnesses?

Mood swings are often a natural part of an outdoor survival situation when people are tired or under pressure, so be cautious about making snap diagnoses and possibly alienating a member of your group. However, displays of uncharacteristic behaviour among your party members may well signal that it is time to stop and rest, giving everyone physical and mental rest and recuperation.

Use the AVPU scale again

Beyond changes of personality, there are deteriorations in consciousness which can lead to full unconsciousness, a condition that should always be taken very seriously. Unconsciousness occurs when the normal patterns of brain activity are interrupted and can result in minor disorders, such as a fainting fit, or major brain damage or respiratory/circulatory failure. In Chapter Two we introduced the AVPU scale, and it is worth repeating this once more:

A = Alert The casualty is fully conscious, aware of his position, and is able to interact fully with the outside world. The diagnostic process for this is simply that you can interact with the person as usual.
V = Voice At this level of consciousness, the casualty is still responding to your voice, though they may be sluggish or incoherent. To test this level of response, give the person simple commands to follow such as getting them to blink their eyes or squeeze your hand if they can hear you.
P = Pain Here the casualty will only seem to respond to pain. Try inducing particularly

sensitive pains or sensations, such as squeezing the ear lobe or scratching the soles of the feet. If the person tries to pull away or they move, then there is still activity being processed between the nerves, spinal cord, and brain.

U = Unresponsive This is a very serious state in which the casualty is totally unconscious, and does not react to any form of stimulus.

Defining a casualty against this scale enables you to make a judgement as to the seriousness of the casualty's condition, but in all categories you should make regular checks of the casualty's vital signs. This is imperative if the casualty is fully unconscious, as a person in this condition is prone to asphyxiation through airway obstruction (by vomit or tongue), and may become unconscious due to problems with circulation, breathing and hydration. As you start to deliver treatment, repeat the AVPU diagnosis continually; this will give you a good indication of whether your treatment is working.

Other general rules for dealing with a fully unconscious person are:

● An unconscious person has weakened body systems, so do not move them roughly or make them sit up unless necessary. This is also important because the person's unconsciousness may be caused by a spinal injury.

● Never give an unconscious person anything whatsoever to eat or drink, as they may choke.

● Keep talking to an unconscious person as he or she may still be able to hear you, and do not say anything to alarm them.

● Remember that the unconscious casualty has lost his or her usual ability to respond to heat, cold, and other climatic phenomenon. You will have to protect them from these, especially in very cold environments where hypothermia is a possibility.

● The casualty should never be left alone when unconscious as his or her condition could change at any moment.

The basic principal to follow with an unconscious casualty is to fully examine them for injuries or illnesses that may be sources of the unconsciousness. These should then be treated in their own right, and consciousness monitored as part of a successful response to treatment. However, any loss of consciousness, whatever the duration, should be treated with concern. We shall now turn to a more specific range of ailments and accidents that can directly impair consciousness, and assess the different responses, including evacuation.

Concussion

Concussion results when a sudden head impact shakes the brain within the skull. The action of shaking alone or the impact of the brain against the wall of the skull can result in a momentary or partial loss of consciousness (the equivalent of the boxer's knockout). While the casualty is unconscious, place them in the recovery position and monitor all the vital signs. When the casualty comes to, they may experience a bad headache and a confused mental state while they recover. Generally they will recover from concussion. Your treatment as a first aider will be mostly proprietary if they come round quickly (within three minutes). Simply keep them rested and warm but under careful observation, as some seemingly minor head injuries can deteriorate unexpectedly.

Warning bells should also start sounding in your mind if the casualty has any of the following symptoms: further loss or impairment of consciousness; persistent vomiting; inability either to concentrate or to remember incidents that happened only a short time ago; an actual skull injury or severe fatigue. If any of these occur then evacuation procedures should begin. Indeed, any

Types of brain injury

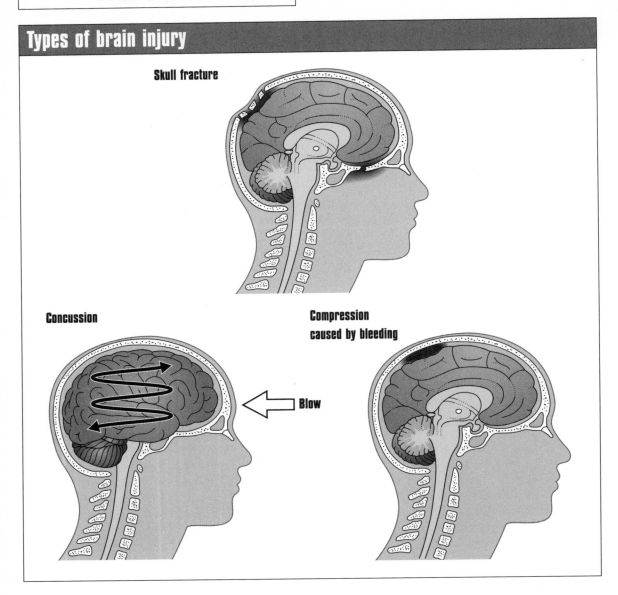

Skull fracture

Concussion

Compression caused by bleeding

Blow

substantial loss of unconsciousness should lead to the evacuation of the person from the field – especially if he or she is unconscious for more than three minutes.

Skull fracture and cerebral compression

A skull fracture is a crack or break in the bone of the skull. Sometimes this can be invisible to the eye of the first aider. The skull may have hairline fractures, which will provide little or no external evidence, though look for more obvious indicators such as any severe bruising or wounds on the skull (remember to search through the hair). Alternatively, there may be a depressed fracture in which a section of the skull is literally smashed inwards. Both types of fracture are very serious and require urgent medical treatment, particularly in the latter case. A depressed fracture compresses the brain either by direct bony fragments or as the result either of bleeding or reactive swelling; there is also a risk of infection from bacteria entering the skull cavity.

Such an injury will be fairly obvious. The casualty will most likely have a bloody, soft depression in the scalp, and they will frequently be unconscious or steadily becoming that way (keep their progress charted using your AVPU scale). For an indication of possible brain injury, see if they have: fluid or blood leaking from the nose or ear; blood leaking into the white of the eye; asymmetry in the position of the face or body.

Cerebral compression is a serious impairment of consciousness, usually the result of a head injury. As its name suggest, this condition is a literal compression of the brain, and it is caused by either the brain swelling from injury and pressing against the skull wall, or by blood accumulating between the skull and the brain and causing a build-up of pressure. In both cases, the effects on consciousness may be dramatic and acutely serious, though be aware that they may not develop immediately after an accident, but take a few hours to manifest. The symptoms of cerebral compression can be:

- A marked abnormality in mental alertness or behaviour, and drifting towards unconsciousness;
- Respiratory difficulty;
- A slow pulse;
- Sudden convulsions or seizures;
- Dilated pupils or pupils of unequal size (if not accompanied by other symptoms of cerebral compression, this could be an indicator, however, of eye problems such as glaucoma);

- A paralysis or weakness down one side of the face or body.

The causes and symptoms of both skull fracture and cerebral compression have been dealt with together because the first aid treatment for these is effectively the same. There is no direct, intrusive method of dealing with damage to the brain itself, so you must set up a rigorous system for monitoring the casualty's vital signs.

Be honest

You must also be prepared to deliver any resuscitation or life support as necessary. This of course means treating any head wounds for bleeding (see Chapter Four). If there is bleeding or fluid loss from the ear, place the casualty in the recovery position, with the injured ear lowest to the ground. Cover the ear with a sterile pad, secured by a bandage, to prevent the ingress of infection.

Dealing with a casualty with brain damage, sadly, can end in death in the context of a survival situation. Techniques such as CPR have no effect on a casualty with acute cerebral injuries to significant parts of the brain, but airway control is vital and rehydration may be required.

In this situation, blunt honesty is also required on the part of the first aider. You must accept you can only do so much.

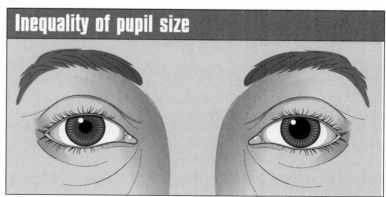

Inequality of pupil size

Applying a head bandage

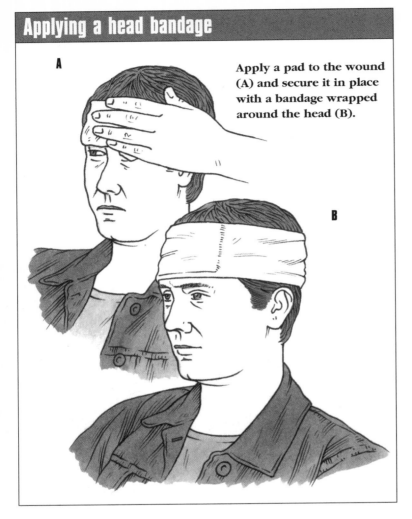

Apply a pad to the wound (A) and secure it in place with a bandage wrapped around the head (B).

Stroke

One in five of us will die of a stroke. Strokes tend to afflict older people or those who suffer from conditions such as high blood pressure. Yet a stroke can happen at any age and is a sudden and debilitating disease. A stroke disrupts or impairs the blood supply to a specific area of the brain. This type of impairment could include a thrombosis – a clot in the cerebral arteries which cuts off blood flow to part of the brain, or a haemorrhage caused by a bleeding artery which floods a section of the brain with blood. In either case, the results are serious and result in either the malfunction of a certain area of the brain or the damage of that area through oxygen deprivation.

The symptoms of stroke vary according to severity, but can include some or all of the following:

● A sudden collapse into unconsciousness with respiratory difficulty. Alternatively, the descent into unconsciousness may be a gradual one over several hours.
● A reddish complexion and a slow, thumping pulse.
● Loss of mental abilities – the casualty will be confused and distressed, and may possibly lose the ability to speak coherently.
● Loss of control over certain bodily functions – one side of the body may become weak or paralysed (look especially at the face and hands), they are unable to move their limbs, the ability to swallow is impaired (thus the individual can often start to dribble), the functions of the bowel and bladder can become involuntary.
● The pupil of one eye may be bigger than the other (read this in context of other symptoms).

One of your primary first aid treatments with a stroke casualty is to make sure that their airway is clear and that they are breathing. This is especially important as those afflicted by stroke may lose control over their airway through a lack of ability to swallow. This is why no food or drink should be given to a stroke casualty. If rescue is a very long time in arriving, there may be exceptions to this rule, but try to avoid it at all costs.

Monitor the casualty's vital signs every ten minutes, but place them in the recovery position if unconscious. If they are conscious, lie them down with their head slightly higher than the feet. Turn the head to one side to allow any saliva to flow out of the mouth rather than down onto the chest. Keep them warm and reassured by your presence.

Convulsions and seizures

Convulsions and seizures can be some of the most alarming ailments a first aider has to treat. They range from a sudden shaking and loss of general awareness, to major contortions of movement and unconsciousness. All convulsions have the same cause – a disruption of the electrical patterns of activity in the brain – but their primary origin can vary. Epilepsy is the perhaps the most common source of convulsions, but other sources include fevers, dehydration, poisoning, meningitis, malaria of the brain, oxygen deprivation, or head injury.

The symptoms of convulsions and seizures vary with the scale of the attack. At one end of the scale, we have a patient who might suddenly go blank and unresponsive, with staring eyes, jerking limbs and strange facial expressions or noises. They could well be on their feet during this state, but they will be unresponsive to

your voice. At the other end of the scale, the casualty may become instantly unconscious, drop to the ground and go rigid, then become convulsed by erratic, violent movements. In this condition, their jaw may clamp rigidly shut (sometimes biting the tongue or lips in the process), they may release their bladder and bowel contents, and they might also stop breathing for the period of the convulsion, which produces a blue-grey coloration in the face.

Seizures by their nature tend to pass after a period of time, but however well the person recovers, it is probably best to move them to evacuation before you (and if you) continue. As a first aider your biggest problem is knowing the cause of the seizure rather than the mechanisms of the seizure, and this can be hard to determine if there is no obvious cause and the person has no record of epilepsy. However, your priority is

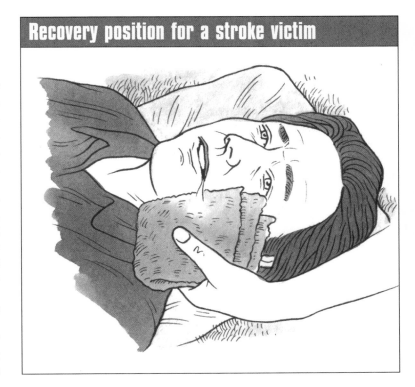

Recovery position for a stroke victim

Tending to a seizure victim

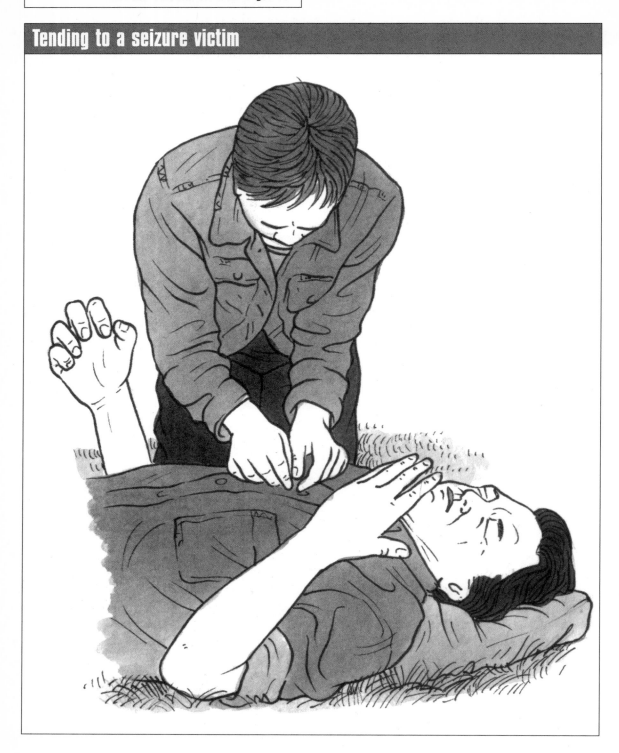

simple treatment to protect the casualty while they are in their fit, and there are fairly straightforward procedures.

While the person is in convulsion or seizure, your full priority is preventing them from harming themselves. This means clearing a safe area around them so that they do not either strike themselves against hard, sharp or hot objects, or preventing them from walking off somewhere where there is danger, a cliff edge for instance. Loosen the clothing around their throat to aid breathing, and place a pad of material (such as a folded jacket or towel) under their head to stop them banging it against the floor. In times past, it was said that something should be put into the casualty's mouth to stop them from biting their tongue – do NOT do this, it increases the chances of the casualty suffocating on a foreign body. Also, do not put your fingers in the patient's mouth – they will be bitten. If the person is not breathing, do not initially try and start resuscitation while they are in the convulsion – their breathing should start again within a short period of time. Yet if respiration is ceased for more than about two minutes, then begin your standard life support procedures.

The convulsion should stop itself after a period of time, though the person's behaviour can continue to be odd for some time, and they may have little recollection of the fit. Sit with the person and talk calmingly to them. They may well want to sleep, and if your situation allows, then let them do so. However, monitor their vital signs, and be aware that further seizures could visit as part of a pattern. When they do finally gain their feet, watch out that they do not harm themselves through clouded thought processes.

Problems with blood-sugar levels

The problems of blood-sugar levels are most commonly associated with the illness diabetes mellitus, in which the body is not able to regulate the amount of glucose in the blood. This can result in either hyperglycaemia, an excess of sugar in the blood, or the reverse, hypoglycaemia, too little sugar in the blood. Both conditions are serious and can result in a potentially life-threatening reduction in consciousness and respiration, but they are generally long-term conditions of which people are aware and are thus controllable through a process of diet and medication. People vulnerable to hyperglycaemia often carry insulin injections or tablets (insulin is the hormone produced in the pancreas which regulates blood-sugar levels), while people prone to hypoglycaemia often carry sugary snacks or glucose tablets to raise their blood-sugar levels when necessary. Nevertheless, it is not that unusual to come across a case of diabetes-related unconsciousness, especially when the casualty loses possession of their medication or if they are taken unawares by an attack. (If going on an expedition with a diabetic, make sure they take more than enough medication with them in case the expedition goes on longer than intended.) In addition, problems of blood-sugar levels may not necessarily be attached to a condition of diabetes.

Blood-sugar problem symptoms

Both hyperglycaemia and hypoglycaemia can lead to a comatose condition and death if left untreated, but their symptoms can vary. Hyperglycaemia (caused by too much insulin) can produce a dramatic thirst, and then advance to rapid respiration, dry skin, a fast pulse, and distinctive smell of acetone on the breath. This can then lead to unconsciousness and coma. Hypoglycaemia expresses itself in fatigue and odd behaviour, a sweaty and clammy complexion and decreasing levels of consciousness and respiration. It is also accompanied by tremors.

In both conditions, when the stage of unconsciousness is reached, then your priority is to perform the analysis of vital signs, and to deliver essential life support as and when required. If at this point the casualty is still conscious, you should help them to take their medication as appropriate, though if a condition such as diabetes is present in your party, then you should have been briefed before you set out on the correct application of the medicine in an emergency. Hyperglycaemia is perhaps the worst of the two conditions in that without insulin and intravenous fluids there is little you can do to directly alleviate the problem. Rapid evacuation is the absolute priority. For a hypoglycaemic casualty who is still conscious, rest and sugary food or drink substances (chocolate, biscuits, sweet tea) can bring an exceptional improvement in the condition very quickly. Even if this is so, evacuation is still recommended, though you will perhaps be able to do this without the call to professional rescue personnel.

Altitude sickness

Altitude sickness is simply caused by the reduction in oxygen levels present at altitudes above 2400m (8000ft), the reduction in air pressure meaning that the oxygen perfusion of the blood through the lungs becomes less efficient and less oxygen becomes available in the bloodstream. This elicits an accelerated respiration rate as the exposed person tries to compensate, but this in turn can disrupt the body's chemical balance and result in the symptoms below.

Increased altitudes can be negotiated by a proper programme of acclimatization (this particularly applies to climbers). Be aware of the altitude of your destination before you set out, and also understand that the further towards the poles from the equator you go, the greater the oxygen deprivation. Take oxygen with you; use it when appropriate or if symptoms of altitude sickness appear. Allow extra time for a journey through high-altitude environments because energy resources will be quickly exhausted. Also plan acclimatization periods. Altitude sick-

ness tends to appear about six hours to four days after arrival at high altitude, but spending two to five days at that altitude usually sees the body stabilize itself in relation to the new environment. Repeat this process as you ascend to new altitudes. Also do not over-exert at high altitudes as this can accelerate more serious conditions of altitude sickness.

The two main forms of altitude sickness are High Altitude Cerebral Edema (HACE) and High Altitude Pulmonary Edema (HAPE). HACE is caused by the swelling of the brain tissue under the effects of oxygen deprivation, while HAPE is a product of capillary fluid being forced into the alveoli of the lungs by the increased pressure of an overworked circulatory system. The symptoms of these conditions are described below, presented from the mildest to the most serious.

HACE
- Headache and nausea; fatigue; unsettled mental state with a tendency towards insomnia; giddiness.
- More acute head pain; vomiting.
- Loss of body co-ordination and coherent mobility.
- Reduction in levels of consciousness and awareness, including incoherence and hallucinations.
- Unconsciousness.

HAPE
- Shortness of breath not alleviated by rest.
- Coughing, including the production of pinkish sputum. This starts with a dry cough at first.
- Congested and difficult breathing with indications of cyanosis; distress.
- Severe respiratory problems and a drop in levels of unconsciousness; casualty may appear pneumonic.
- Unconsciousness and respiratory failure.

HACE in its earliest forms is not serious, and is simply an indication of adjustment to altitude. Giving non-prescription pain medication (if a headache is present) and plenty of rest are what is needed here. Avoid sedatives. However, for mild to severe forms of HACE or any evidence at all of HAPE, more decisive action is needed. Naturally, the fact that both conditions are caused by high altitude means that a first aider's initial actions should be to stabilize the immediate problems as needed, and then rapidly get the patient to a lower altitude. Care should be taken in this as the casualty's weakened body systems should not be over-exerted or the problem might be exacerbated. Descents of just 500m (1640ft) can start to make a difference in the condition, but if the problems are significant aim to descend about 600–1200m (2000–4000 feet). A temporary alternative is to use the barometric pressure bags available to climbers. The casualty is sealed inside the bag, then oxygen is pumped in to replicate a higher barometric pressure. Use this only to get the patient stabilized and then make the descent. With HAPE, keep monitoring respiration and be prepared to support or resuscitate along conventional lines. Keep descending, and get the casualty to professional medical support.

Intoxication

Drunkenness is perhaps one of the most commonly experienced causes of altered consciousness. In an outdoor survival situation, severe drunkenness can cause respiratory failure and make the casualty more vulnerable to hypothermia. The symptoms of drunkenness include: mental incoherence, a smell of alcohol on the breath and through the skin, inability to move sensibly, a severe personality change. Make sure through a historical diagnosis that the person is drunk; some serious conditions such as head injuries have been mistaken for intoxication.

A greater cause for concern is if the casualty starts to lapse into periods of unconsciousness. You should place them in the recovery position to stop potential choking on their own vomit, and monitor their vital signs regularly. Keep them warm to prevent a hypothermic response to the environment.

Extreme stress reaction

One of the primary causes of an altered state of consciousness is stress, and in a survival situation the first aider may experience an extreme stress reaction either personally or at second hand.

When faced with a dangerous or alarming situation, the brain's hypothalamus triggers hormonal reactions which release adrenaline and noradrenaline from the adrenal medulla into the bloodstream. The results are an increase in respiration, heart rate, and blood pressure, and blood is drawn away from surface vessels and the brain and diverted to the muscles to fuel their efforts. After this initial physiological reaction, hormonal levels tend to stabilize themselves though the psychology of the person remains acutely focused.

The problem with an extreme stress reaction is that we are unaccustomed to it (the reaction is a very ancient one which we tend not to use regularly). Mental impotence and freezing can be induced by the unfamiliar sensations occurring in the body, and the casualty may exhibit symptoms of shock as the blood drains to the muscles.

Psychological confusion, a retreat from reality, and physical weakness can occur, and the first aider will need to take control of the situation to ensure the sufferer does not endanger themselves.

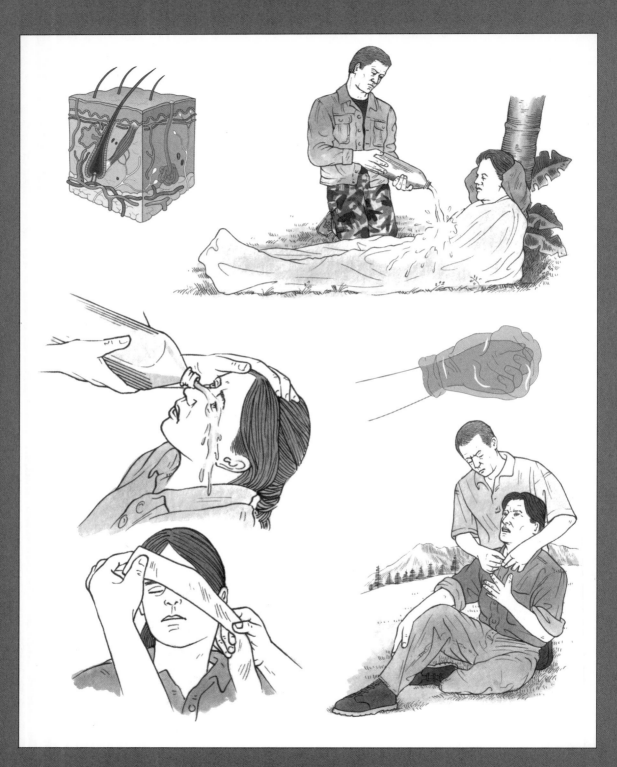

CHAPTER SIX

Burns & scalds

Burns, especially if they are serious, can be among the most traumatic wounds a first aider may have to deal with. Whatever their cause, burns can inflict great pain and damage on the human body.

The dangers of receiving burns are possibly greater in a survival or outdoor scenario than in a domestic situation. Outdoor pursuits often involve open, hand-tended fires and barbecues, tins of boiling water balanced on small Primus stoves, and the carriage of various mechanisms and fuel for producing fire and heat.

From the first aider's point of view, burns can range across the full spectrum of emergency challenge. At one end of the scale there are the minor burns we have all encountered – touching a hot cooking pot, a slight rope burn, contact with the end of a cigarette.

At the other end of the scale are full-depth burns covering a high percentage of the casualty's body. These may not only cause direct heat and flame damage, but also have life-threatening repercussions through fluid loss and ancillary injuries such as smoke inhalation.

Thus as we go through the first aid treatment for burns, it is important to remember

Sources of burns

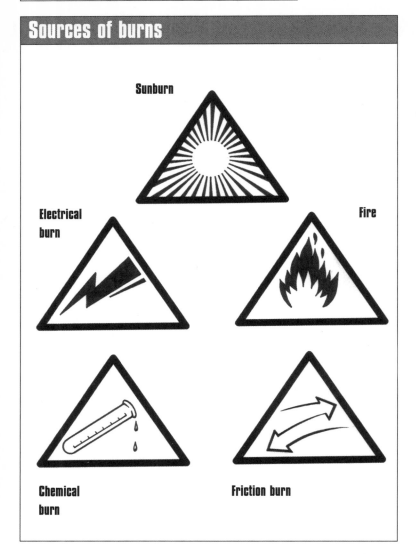

Sunburn

Electrical burn

Fire

Chemical burn

Friction burn

the authenticity of the real thing, but adjusting to the sight of it will be excellent training should you have to deal with a serious burn in real life.

BURNS AND THE HUMAN SKIN

Burns have many different and diverse causes, all resulting in injury when destructive levels of heat come in contact with a point on the human body. In fact, the list of burn causes is surprisingly broad, and goes well beyond contact with flame. The main types of burns in an outdoor survival situation are:

- **Dry burn** – contact with a direct dry heat source such as a flame, hotplate, or cigarette.
- **Friction burn** – burn caused by heat build-up through friction, most commonly a rope burn.
- **Sunburn** – over-exposure to the sun's ultra-violet rays.
- **Scald** – caused by high-temperature liquid or steam.
- **Cold burn** – often not considered a burn, but frostbite or contact with freezing metals of substances can cause burn injuries.
- **Electrical burn** – less common in the outdoors, but still possible from sources such as lightning or overhead pylons.
- **Chemical burns** – can come from acid or alkali substances, and a wide variety of industrial chemicals.
- **Respiratory burns** – burns to the mouth, nose, windpipe, or lungs through

that any significant burn impacts on the whole body system, and the casualty must be treated accordingly. The other thing to remember is that treating serious burns can be a psychologically disturbing experience. The casualty may be screaming with the great pain that often accompanies burns, and the sight and smell of scorched flesh can be particularly nauseating. Ideally, attend a first aid training centre where burns injuries are replicated using make-up. This will not have the inhalation of superheated air or caustic gases.

We shall consider the treatments for these burns each in turn, but first we must understand how the human skin is structured, and then we must examine the mechanism through which it is damaged by burns of varying intensity.

Human skin is composed of two layers. The outermost layer, the visible part in contact with the outside world, is called the epidermis and acts as a protective waterproof layer. Beneath this is the dermis, the major part of the human skin. The dermis contains nerves, muscles, sweat glands, and the roots of the hair follicles, which terminate in or through the epidermis. Finally, there is a layer of fat tissue beneath and separate to the dermis. This layer supplies the skin with vital nutrients.

Keep in mind that the skin is an organ – in fact, the body's largest. Its functions are protective and regulatory: it protects against infections and injuries from the outside world, while also helping to regulate body temperature. The skin can control heat loss or retention by constricting or dilating blood capillaries at its surface. It also performs this function through controlling perspiration and shivering.

When treating a burn, the information you are looking for to guide your first aid actions is:

- How deep is the burn?
- How much of the body is the burn covering?

The depth of burns is judged according to three distinct levels – first degree, second degree, and third degree.

- **First degree** – No significant damage is done to the skin, and there is no structural impairment of the nerves or blood vessels. This includes superficial burns such as sunburn, and the characteristics are redness, swelling, surface pain, or sensitivity. This should require little or no treatment.
- **Second degree** – Here the epidermis is damaged, but the blood vessels and nerves beneath are not significantly affected. Second degree burns usually result in blistering, pain, swelling, and the necessity for some level of medical

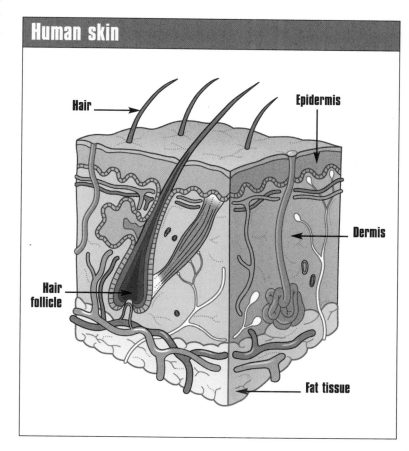

Human skin

Hair

Epidermis

Dermis

Hair follicle

Fat tissue

treatment. They are, however, serious enough to be life-threatening if they cover more than 60 per cent of the body surface.

- **Third degree** – The most serious category of burn, in which the burn damages both layers of the skin including nerves, blood vessels, and even the underlying fat tissue. Bone and muscle may be visible. These burns are very severe, and may be charred black or grey or waxy in appearance.

Each of these three burn types has a different healing response. After burning, blood vessels leak fluid into the site as a repair mechanism. This fluid either forms into blisters, or gathers on the skin surface. Major burns send the victim into severe volume shock through the sheer amount of fluid loss.

An additional problem is that the damage inflicted to the skin through burns makes the casualty acutely vulnerable to infection. This can be a major complication if there is some time between injury and professional attention. As a technique of diagnosis, try pricking the area of the burn with a needle. If the casualty feels pain then the burn is superficial; if they don't, then the burn has penetrated more deeply and equals a third degree burn.

So how do we judge the level of burn? We have already described the degree of burn, but the other measure is the extent of burn coverage on the human body. This factor allows the first aider to judge the extent of fluid loss, and thus the danger of shock developing. Each area of the human body can be mapped out into respective percentages of total body area, and usefully works in multiples of nines:

- **Head:** 9 per cent;
- **Front of torso:** 18 per cent;
- **Back of torso:** 18 per cent;
- **Arms:** 9 per cent each;
- **Genital area:** 1 per cent;
- **Front of legs:** 9 per cent each;
- **Back of legs:** 9 per cent each;
- **Feet and hands:** 1 per cent each.

Armed with the ability to diagnose both extent and depth of burns, you should now be able to judge the seriousness of burns suffered in an accident. The following are guidelines for response:

- Professional medical treatment is required for a second degree burn of one per cent or more of the body surface, and any third degree burn over any percentage;
- Shock will ensue from any second degree burn over 10 per cent of the body surface area;
- Respiratory burns should be treated as a possible cause of life-threatening injury.
- Burns over 60 per cent of an adult's body surface incur a high risk of fatality if professional medical help is not received;
- Burns are especially serious if they occur alongside another type of injury;
- The young and old are particularly vulnerable to adverse burn response.

Procedure for dealing with burns

We will now explore specific treatments for different types of burn injury. However, underlying almost all the techniques outlined below are a common set of procedures.

Firstly, the source of the burn must be controlled, extinguished, or removed. If the casualty is on fire, wrap him or her tightly in an item of clothing, or roll them on the ground to extinguish the flames. Remove combustible materials from the site of a fire. Make sure a sunburn victim is out of direct sunlight. Whatever the case, remove the casualty and yourself from further danger either by safely negating the source of the burn, or by getting away from it. Remember, that fire needs access to oxygen (which is prohibited by smothering flames) and fuel to burn. Try to cut off both of these sources by whatever means possible.

Secondly, take the temperature out of the burn. Burns can take some time to do their damage, and residual heat in the burn area can keep damaging body tissue for hours if the heat is not controlled, especially if clothing still traps the heat on the burn site. Pour copious amounts of cold water over a burn, and keep this up for at least 10 minutes (or use packs of snow in a cold climate). Submerge a burnt limb in a flowing stream or river, though using sterilized water sources are better because burn injuries are particularly vulnerable to infection. You will have an indication that a burn is properly cooled if stopping the irrigation does not increase the casualty's pain. Once a burn is thoroughly cooled, dressings can be applied as described below. One cautionary note, however. Do not cool the casualty to such an extent that hypothermia becomes a risk. Victims of serious burns are particularly vulnerable because the skin's ability to regulate temperature is impaired.

Thirdly, fluids should be given to the casualty partly to counteract the fluid loss he or she has already suffered. Fluids should be given frequently in small doses, preferably cold drinks, and certainly no alcohol. Adding half a teaspoon of salt to a pint of water also helps the casualty replenish lost salt content.

Finally, it should go without saying that you must regularly check the patient's vital signs, especially if the burns are serious. Keep a close eye on the development of symptoms for shock (see Chapter Three), and any subsequent respiratory or cardiac

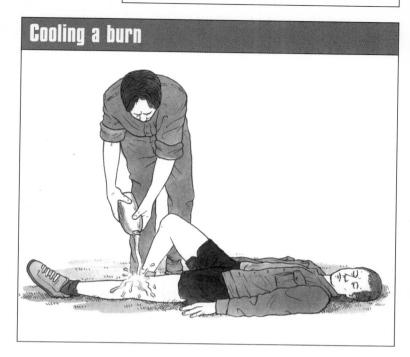

Cooling a burn

failure. Especially if the casualty has been burned by fire, assume respiratory burning, and check that the airway is clear and that breathing is normal.

Major burns and scalds

With any major burn or scald (second or third degree, with significant body coverage for the type), the immediate priority is to remove or extinguish the source of the burn, then lay the casualty down. Outdoors, sanitary practices may be difficult, but try to keep the burn area from direct contact with the ground. Then start pouring cold liquid directly onto the burn site. If you can, remove any watches, rings, belts, ropes, boots, and clothing from affected areas, as subsequent swelling may make them difficult to remove and they may restrict blood supply to the area. Clothing can be carefully cut or peeled away from the wound, but do not attempt to remove clothing which is sticking. Instead pour water directly onto the material, and keep it soaked and cold (at the

Protecting a burnt hand in a bag

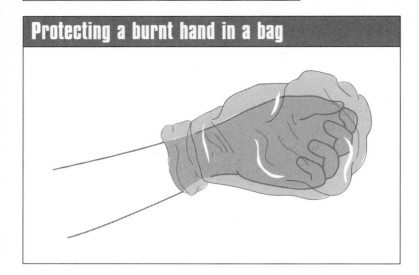

should you apply any ointments or fats to the burned region – the old wives' tale about using butter to treat a burn is positively dangerous.

Respiratory burns

Around one in five people who suffer from respiratory burns dies from them, such is the seriousness of the injury. Respiratory burns occur with the inhalation of superheated gas (including air) or steam. The result is that lungs and airways blister and swell, with fluid building up in the lungs and threatening to drown the casualty. Signs of respiratory burns include external burns and swelling around the face, redness inside the mouth, a swollen tongue, soot gathering around the nose and mouth, sooty sputum, and obvious respiratory difficulty.

Respiratory burns are difficult for the first aider to treat. The initial step is to give the casualty as much access to fresh air as possible. Remove them from the site of smoke or fumes, and relax any constricting clothing such as helmet straps or tight coat collars. Give the casualty sips of cold water to try to control swelling, but be careful as the burn may have affected their ability to swallow effectively. Be vigilant about the casualty's respiratory rate and condition, and prepare to deliver artificial respiration if need be. Maintain this vigilance over the entire period until evacuation, as the pulmonary fluids will build up as the lungs attempt their healing process.

Chemical burns

Chemical burns are unusual in an outdoor setting, mainly because you are generally well away from the industrialized locations where chemicals are concentrated.

same time, remembering the caution about hypothermia).

After a period of cooling, you should dress the wound to reduce the possibility of infection through bacteria. Do not dress a burn as you would a bleeding wound. Instead, simply cover the area with a sterile dressing or any piece of clean material which is non-fluffy. Only secure this material if the wind is removing it or the affected part of the body is awkward. Burnt hands or feet can be loosely wrapped in plastic bags which are secured at the wrist or ankle, though as with all dressings for burns, do not secure them directly onto the skin. While skin around the burns area may seem unaffected, it may rapidly change in an hour or two. If a hand or foot is burnt, separate each digit with individual dressings before bandaging to stop rubbing and sticking.

Once these procedures have been completed you should then concentrate on looking out for the visible symptoms of shock or respiratory distress. Do not interfere in any way with the burn injury itself, unless there are smouldering pieces of material in it which need to be removed. Blisters should never be burst as this can introduce infection into the site of the wound. Neither

However, this is not always the case. In certain developing countries or those with poor environmental control, such as Russia, chemicals can be encountered in streams and rivers in high concentrations (do not bathe in a water system which has a significant number of death fish floating on its surface). Furthermore, certain expeditions may have to carry chemicals or solvents for scientific purposes.

Chemical burns are as serious as thermal burns mainly because a chemical reaction can be much more resistant to irrigation (washing with water), and can keep up its burning process for many hours. Symptoms can include the presence of a chemical source, a rash, blistering, peeling or general discoloration of the skin, and a burning type of pain.

Treatment

The treatment for a chemical burn is essentially the same as that for a thermal burn – remove affected clothing, wash with water, monitor respiration and airway closely. However, you should wash the area for longer, and a minimum of 20 minutes is recommended. Some things not to do are: do not attempt any chemical neutralization of acid with alkali or vice versa unless you very clearly know what you are doing from specific training; do not put yourself in a direct skin-to-skin contact with the casualty, and

use a face mask or some other improvised protection if giving artificial respiration. Try to find out which chemical is involved, as such information will be useful later.

If a chemical has been in contact with the eye, you will notice symptoms such as the

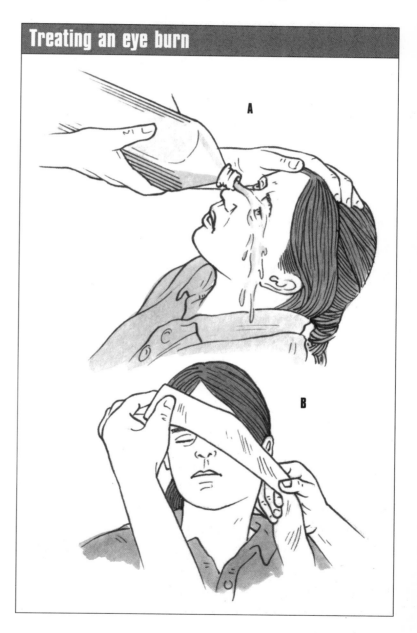

Treating an eye burn

swelling and watering of the eye, an inability to open the eye, and a report of severe eye pain. Keep the casualty's hands, and your own, away from the eye, but irrigate it under cold water for about 10 minutes, gently opening the eyelid to ensure a thorough washing. Make sure that the eye you are washing is lower than the other to prevent cross contamination from the water, and do not let any water flow across the casualty's mouth. Once this is completed, cover the eye with a pad of clean dressing, or better an eye pad which should be in your first aid kit.

Electrical burns

From an outdoor point of view, the main dangers from electricity are lightning strike or contact with high-voltage power lines (which can be found in even the most remote of places.) Burns caused by these powerful electrical sources are not necessarily the greatest danger to the casualty, though they can generate serious third-degree injuries. A lightning strike or other high-voltage shock disrupts the nervous impulses, and the casualty usually dies from heart stoppage. However, if fatality does not ensue, then you should prepared to treat significant burns and shock.

Despite their awesome multi-million volt power, lightning shocks only kill about one in five of their victims, and tend not to leave major burns. This is because the lightning flash only lasts about 1000th of a second, unlike a severe domestic electrocution which can last many seconds and can transfer a great deal of heat. However, the massive detonation that lightning makes can often kill through inflicting internal damage by smashing tissue and bone like a hammer.

Lightning can strike a person both by direct hit and also by a near hit, which sends currents of electricity coursing through the ground and up into the body. Electricity only harms the human body if there is a point of entry and a point of exit, so if you come across a lightning casualty, they will probably have major third-degree burns at two distinct points (with lightning most often the shoulder and the leg/foot). The casualty may also be unconscious, suffering from shock and deafened by a lightning blast (so they may not be able to respond to your voice). Apart from the deafness, high-voltage electrical shocks from both industrial and domestic sources will have the same symptoms to greater or lesser extent.

The treatment for lightning or high-voltage electrical shock is the same. In both cases think very seriously about rescuing your colleague if the source of electricity is still present – lightning that has just struck in

General principles for lightning safety

- If lightning is evident, keep away from high ground, and isolated, or otherwise very tall, natural features (such as trees, boulders, and landmass).
- Keep away from large metal objects, and if possible put aside metal objects you are carrying (but do not if you could lose valuable equipment).
- If you are caught out in lightning, lie as flat as you can on the ground; preferably place some dry insulating material beneath you, such as a coiled rope.
- If you feel your skin tingling, it is very likely that you are about to be struck by lightning. If you are not lying flat, very quickly fall to a hands and knees position, as your arms may conduct the worst of the current down to the ground.

one place can easily strike again, and high-voltage electricity can arc out from its source without direct contact. Only if you are sure there is no danger to yourself or others should the casualty be brought in. Immediately check pulse and respiration. Particularly after lightning strikes, a heart can start itself after a temporary cessation, but in some cases the casualty will need your full assistance with respiration and circulation. Even once these appear stabilized, keep checking them regularly as the disruptive effects of electrical shock can destabilize the vital systems many hours after the shock occurred.

Treating electrical burns is a similar process to treating any other burn. They must be thoroughly irrigated with water, burnt clothing should be removed, and the injury dressed as described above. Then evacuate.

Sunburn

Sunburn is a very common complaint caused by over-exposure to the sun's radioactive rays. It should not occur amongst experienced outdoors, men and women. Even in the hottest climates, make sure that vulnerable skin is well covered. Modern materials ensure that wearing clothing such as a long-sleeved shirt and a hat will not result in your overheating. Also use a high-factor sun block lotion (Factor 20 and above), even if you have seasoned skin.

Sunburn has varying degrees of severity, and tends to be more serious for fair-skinned

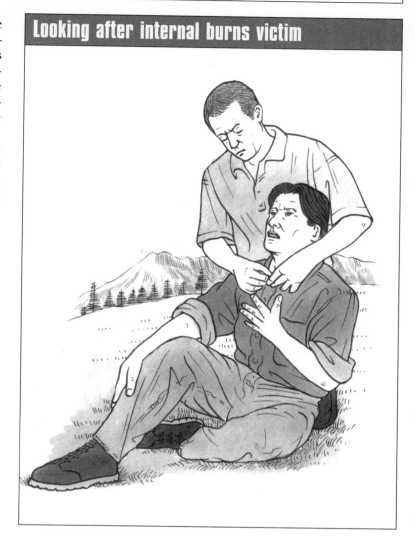

Looking after internal burns victim

persons. It ranges from a light redness and tenderness to the skin, to a deep red and blistered surface. As with all burns, do not burst the blisters, but treat primarily by applying cold compresses (water soaked material applied to the wound and re-drenched regularly to keep it chilled) for around 10 minutes, and also provide the casualty with cold water to drink. Most importantly, make the casualty either into shelter or, if your have to keep moving, covered up with full-length items of clothing. The sun's rays can also

Treatment for large-area body burns

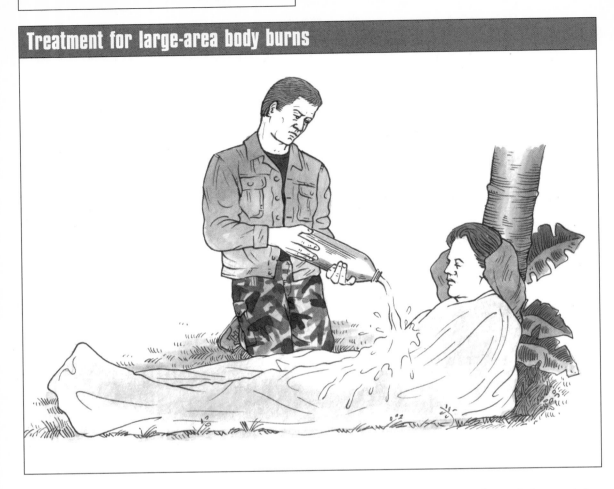

burn the eyes, as they can when reflected off a bright surface such as snow (snow blindness). For treatment of these conditions, and also on cold-created burns, see Chapter Eight.

Friction burns and blisters

Friction burns are of particular danger to the mountain climber, whose ropes may run through hands or around the legs, and generate enough friction heat to produce a substantial burn and deep wound. Prevention is always better than cure, and proper clothing, gloves, and climbing technique should help prevent these injuries. However, if they do occur, the treatment is the generic burns

treatment – irrigate and cool (mountains often have good supplies of snow to hand), cover, and then assess for any other injuries.

Blisters are one form of friction injury which need special consideration. This is not only because they are so tremendously common, but also because if they are left untreated and in insanitary conditions for long, they can produce serious infections.

Prevention of foot blisters, the most common form of blister, is possible through changing socks regularly, wearing properly-fitted boots and performing organized foot checks on a walk. Blisters will announce themselves by producing a recognizable hot spot on your skin, and this is the moment at

General principles for forest fire safety

● Pick your escape route based on travelling into the wind – the wind direction will usually indicate the direction of the fire's travel.

● Even if it gets very hot indeed keep your clothing on as it will protect from burns caused by heated air.

● Stay away from high ground as forest fires burn more quickly when travelling up hill.

● If you have to run through flames, cover as much skin as possible and dampen clothing with water. Hold your breath while passing through the flames, as fast as possible, using a piece of damp cloth to cover your nose and mouth.

which you should take action with a change of footwear or socks. If an ointment is available, it should be applied. Once the area has been cooled and treated, you can set off again.

Sometimes blisters will develop fully, and as with all burns, do not voluntarily burst them. However, with blisters there can be exceptions, especially if the blister is so sited as to affect your mobility. In this case, bursting should be applied through the following technique:

● Clean the area around the blister thoroughly using soap and water which can act as a good enough disinfectant;

● You now need a sterilized needle or blade with which to lance the blister. Sterilization can be achieved by immersing the steel in alcohol, boiling it for about 5 minutes, or holding it over a flame. Even better is to have sterilized needles sealed away in your medical pack;

● Pierce the blister at one end, usually its lowest

point, and allow the fluid to drain out. Do not pull away the blister skin. Instead let it stay there to protect to wound from infection;

● Cover the wound and regularly clean it. Keep checking it for infection and apply some antibiotic ointment if you have it.

Lancing a blister

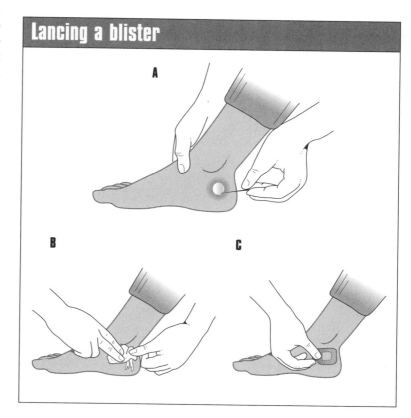

A

B

C

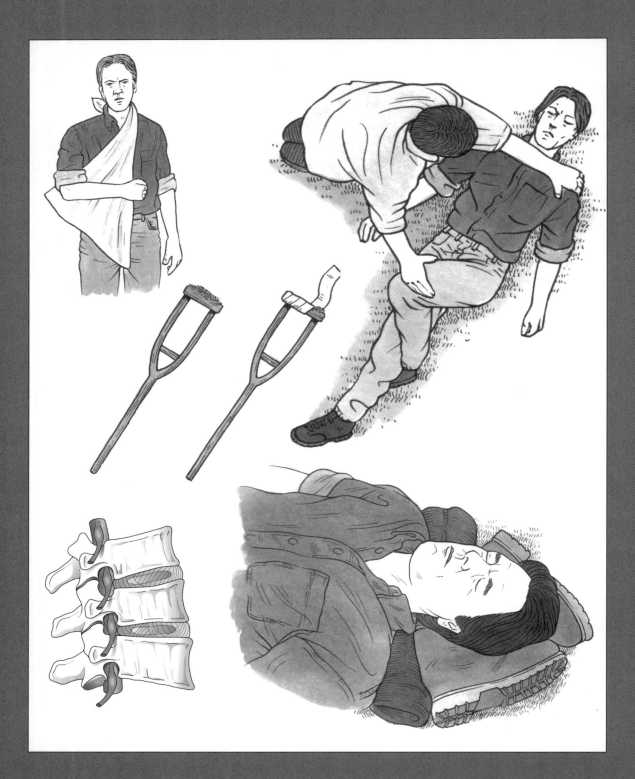

CHAPTER SEVEN

Bone, joint, & muscle injuries

The human skeleton is one of the true miracles of nature. Its intricate structure of interconnecting bones, joints, ligaments, tendons, and muscles not only gives our entire physique a rigid form and shape, but it also enables us to move with great flexibility and freedom of expression.

Yet, although the skeleton is very strong in both its individual parts and overall structure, it is also vulnerable to injury from outside forces. Damage to any of its constituent parts – as those of us who have broken a bone will know – is extremely debilitating and painful. More seriously, particular forms of damage to the skeleton can also impact on the body's respiratory, circulatory, and respiratory systems. This chapter will not only focus on how best to deal with the practicalities of handling local bone breaks and muscle damage, but it will also emphasize that when handling such emergencies, your attention and concern should go first to the patient's overall condition rather than to attending to the immediate injury.

THE MUSCULOSKELETAL SYSTEM

As we all know, the skeleton is made up of bones. Bones are primarily formed from a composition of collagen and calcium phosphate. This combination makes them tough,

The human skeleton

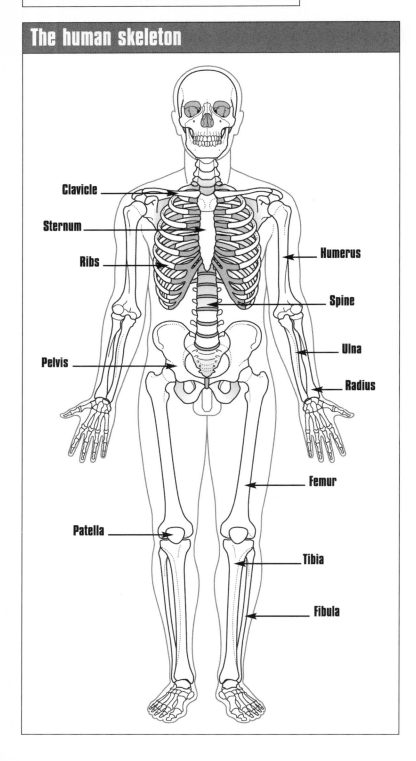

Clavicle

Sternum

Ribs

Humerus

Spine

Pelvis

Ulna

Radius

Femur

Patella

Tibia

Fibula

light, and incredibly strong for their weight. All the bones link together from head to foot to provide the shape and form of the human body. They also provide a protective cage around the vital internal organs of the torso.

Linking the bones together are the joints which allow the skeleton to achieve a range of different movements throughout the body. Joints, like bones, come in several different forms, suited to their local purpose and activity:

- **Ball-and-socket joints** One bone terminates in a ball-like head, which fits into the concave end piece of the adjoining bone. The ball is thus able to rotate in the socket, enabling a swinging motion over a broad arc. Examples of ball-and-socket joints are found in the shoulder and hip.
- **Hinge joints** These are joints which allow the skeleton to perform bending and straightening actions, such as found in the elbow and the knee. Hinge joints have only one plane of movement, which is restricted by the shape of the junction.
- **Movable joints** The spine is a good example of this type of joint, which is made up of bones that rock or glide

across each other, though with nowhere near the same range of movement as the other type of joints.

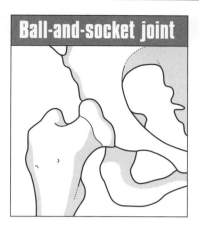

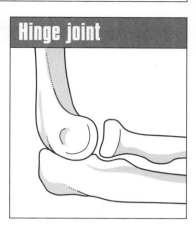

These are the three types of moveable joint in the human body. All of these joints are held in place by ligaments which are bundles of strong fibrous tissue which link bones together. These reach across the adjoining bones, and the friction between the bones as they make these movements is limited by a covering of cartilage across the bone ends.

Of course, the skeletal system as it has been described so far has no animating force behind it. This animating force is provided by the human body's system of muscles. Muscles are contractile tissues that operate either voluntarily or involuntarily. The muscles which flex and power the skeletal system are generally controlled by conscious decision, although they can also be powered by involuntary response when reacting to some painful stimuli. Muscles are connected to the bones by tendons, and in paired configurations give human limbs various possibilities of movement. By working in pairs, with one muscle contracting while the other muscle relaxes, the muscles in the limbs are able to deliver strength of movement in two directions.

Those who engage in vigorous outdoor pursuits are usually much more acquainted with the nature of their musculoskeletal systems than most. However, it is worth bearing in mind that some conditioning of the system is advisable before participating in such outdoor activities. Before setting out on any survival expedition or event, check that no-one has any previous injuries to bones or muscles which might affect the person's

physical competence later. This is particularly important with regards to any recurrent back problems which might surface should any heavy lifting work be required. If you are engaged in rock climbing, canoeing, hiking or similar activities necessitating strong muscle tone and durability, make sure that you have developed the required musculature, preferably by building up your level of participation in the relevant activity.

Furthermore, it is essential to warm up muscles before embarking on any strenuous activity. This means lightly exercising each group of muscles until they are warm and flexible. Before exercise, cold muscles have less pliability and range of motion than warm muscles, and so are more prone to injury. Flexibility is also important; indeed strength is supported by flexible muscles. Even if you are engaged in walking activities, do regular stretching exercises of all your body muscles as this will make the muscles less prone to sprains and strains.

MUSCULOSKELETAL INJURIES AND DIAGNOSIS
Fractures
Bones can take great punishment without incurring damage. This is thanks mainly to their great intrinsic strength and their ability to flex under pressure. However, sometimes the forces exerted on a bone are far too

Fracture types

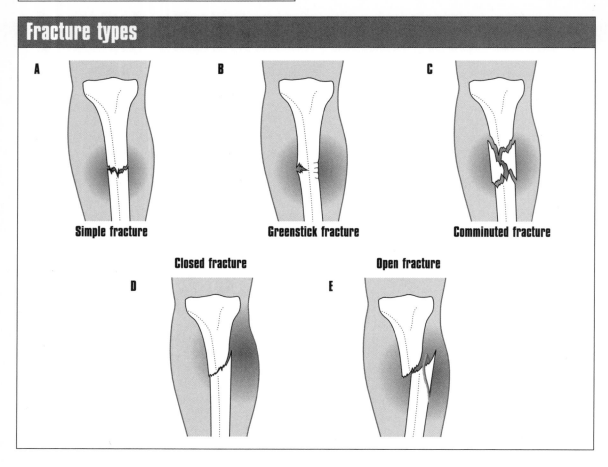

A — Simple fracture

B — Greenstick fracture

C — Comminuted fracture

D — Closed fracture

E — Open fracture

much for it to control. As a result, a fracture occurs. Fractures are usually the result of accidents such as falls, blows, twisting, or over-bending, which take a bone beyond its capabilities for endurance. Thus fractures tend to be more common in sports such as rock climbing, mountain biking, and canoeing. During these sports, accidents at speed or at height tend to lead to impact injuries upon hard surfaces such as rocks and tree stumps.

A fracture is essentially a bone break or crack, and there are several different kinds. Overall they can be defined by whether the break is open or closed. If open (also known as a compound fracture), the bone has broken the surface of the skin and is protruding.

This is usually caused by the bone break creating sharp edges which are then levered or pushed through the skin. In a closed fracture, the break is contained under the skin.

A fracture can also be classified as either stable or unstable. A stable fracture has taken place when the bone is broken, but the broken halves are jammed together by the force of the injury so that the break is not moving. Someone suffering from this type of break may well be in extreme pain, but they will often be able to seemingly use the damaged limb as normal. An unstable fracture means that the bones at the break point are knocked out of line with one another, with some motion resulting between the broken bones.

Within these two categories are two main types of bone break for a grown adult: simple and comminuted. A simple fracture is a straightforward break in which the bone is snapped along a particular angle. A comminuted fracture is messier, and involves the bone shattering into many different bone fragments. From a first aider's point of view, if the fracture is closed you will rarely be able to diagnose the difference between them, though an historical analysis of the cause of the injury may give indicate to you whether the fracture is of the first type or the second.

Diagnosing a fracture

Your primary concern in tending such injuries is not so much the bone itself, but the impact the break has had on vital organs and blood vessels in the proximity of the injury. When bones break they can often form very sharp, spiky edges, and these can pierce tissue and cut arteries and veins when forced through the tissue by the impact of the break. Thus when attending to someone with a suspected fracture, make your initial priority a check of their vital signs, particularly if the fracture is to the femur (thigh bone), pelvis, ribs, spine, or skull. All of these bones if broken can have a profound impact on respiration, circulation, and the nervous system. Bleeding from a broken bone can be internal as well as invisible (for the signs of internal bleeding see Chapter Four), so it is necessary to perform all the regular checks for developing shock.

A general diagnosis of a fracture is easy if the fracture is open, or if it is closed but displaying a marked deformity or unnatural angle. However, the diagnosis is more difficult when the injury is closed and the limb is in line. In this situation, bruising, swelling, and other wounds can mask the break by giving it the appearance of soft tissue wounding.

Your first point of call is to make an historical diagnosis (see Chapter Two). Gather witnesses and find out what happened to the casualty. Assess what impacts or what contortions the person suffered as the accident was taking place, and use your common sense to judge whether this would have been likely to result in a break. Also ask the witnesses whether or not they remember hearing the distinct snapping sound of breakage, a noise which can be quite loud in the case of a breaking arm or leg bone.

Your next step is to inspect the casualty. If the wound is bruised and inflamed, and the casualty is unable to move or put weight on the injury, then a break is likely. The casualty may also report the bones grinding together, or you may detect this by laying your hand on the wound area (do not manipulate the limb to achieve this diagnosis). Check an injured limb against the uninjured one to see if there are differences in contour and shape. The wound will be very painful to the touch. A deeper level of diagnosis involves checking for nerve or circulatory damage.

Pulse and sensation tests

If a limb is damaged, check just beyond the wound site to see if the limb has a pulse, or whether it is turning white or blue. This may indicate that circulation to the extremity has been cut off.

Combine this with sensation tests – tickle the extremity of the damaged limb to see if the casualty can feel it. If not, or if the limb is becoming numb or tingling, then it may be suffering from oxygen deprivation or nerve damage. Both of these conditions can lead to a loss of the limb if they are not rectified.

Your treatment, which will be explored below, is to help the casualty regain his or her circulation, sensation, and movement if possible. However, evacuation or rescue should always be a priority in the event of a significant bone break. If after all your diagnoses, you are unable to decide as to whether the bone is broken or not, assume that it is and treat it accordingly.

Shoulder dislocation

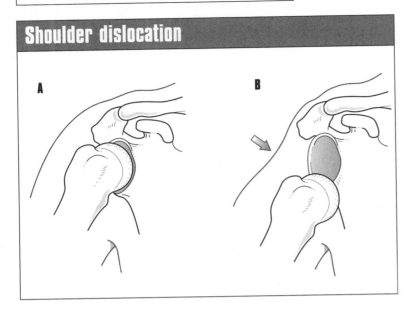

A   B

Dislocations

A dislocation occurs literally where the bones at a joint are forced out of their normal position, either partially or completely. Causes range from blows (though these are a less common source of dislocations) and especially wrenching injuries, to natural muscular exertions such as over-stretching. The diagnosis of this type of injury is essentially the same as that for a fracture with one or two differences.

Naturally, dislocations are in specific locations at the joints, so any visible signs of displacement will be at these specific locations rather than at mid points. There may not be the same bruising if the dislocation is the result of a wrench injury – such as that incurred during a climbing fall in which the drop is arrested by the arm – but nonetheless, inflammation and certainly pain will both be present.

Muscle, tendon, and ligament injuries

Damage to muscles, tendons, and ligaments can be difficult to diagnose with specificity, unless it is caused by an external injury. All three structures can be torn or strained by over-exertion or wrenching, but also through repetitive actions (such as rowing or pedalling) which create an injury through wear-and-tear.

Diagnosis of such injuries will usually be done for you by the casualty – they will report a localized, burning pain which will either limit or prohibit movement. Sometimes this will occur rapidly in conjunction with a particular movement, or build over a period of time. The injury can be accompanied by swelling and redness.

A separate category of muscle injury is bruising which goes deep enough to implicate the muscle tissue. A bruise results from blood escaping from blood vessels torn by a blow and tracking to the skin. There may be associated pain, swelling, and loss of mobility.

TREATING FRACTURES AND DISLOCATIONS

As has already been noted, your first priority when attending a fracture or dislocation casualty is to check their vital signs for any signs of respiratory, circulatory, or nervous system danger. Once this is done, then you can attend to the injury itself.

Your diagnostic tests will have assessed whether the broken or dislocated limb (if a limb it is – they tend to be the most common area of skeletal injury alongside ribs) is suffering from circulatory or nervous deprivation, and you should then proceed to treat along the following generic principles (specific injury sites will be dealt with in due course).

Firstly, stop the casualty from moving around (preferably get them to lie down), and keep the injured area still. If the wound is of the open kind, treat the bleeding as described in Chapter Four, and if you have to dress this type of wound without retracting the bone within the skin (see below), build pads of material around the bone and then bandage these pads in place covering the whole injury site.

Traction

Next your objectives should be to align the bones of the injury site through a process of applying traction. The purpose of traction is to return the broken limb to a more natural alignment by using a pulling and relocation manoeuvre. This would not usually be done in a situation where rescue services were only minutes away. Yet in a survival situation, it is recommended to keep the risk of further tissue damage caused by moving bones to a minimum, and it allows you greater possibilities for moving the casualty without additional damage. It also offers the best option for giving back normal circulation to an injured limb. Exceptions to this are breaks (not dislocations) at joints such as the elbow, finger, and shoulder, and these are best protected by being supported in a position which is the mid point of their normal range of movement.

Traction is performed by gently but firmly pulling the broken limb, first in the direction the bone is pointing then swinging it back in line with the original limb position. Do this slowly over a period of 10–15 minutes or so, keeping the traction on the limb, while at the same time encouraging the casualty to relax his muscles to allow you to draw the

extremity towards you. The point you are aiming for is when the broken ends of the bone are ready to be placed back together in a more natural alignment. Once the limb is fully extended, align it as it should be normally – you can get someone else to do this for maximum accuracy – and then relax your pull.

The bones, muscles, and blood vessels should now be in something approaching their original configuration. This procedure can also be done with open fractures, though you should be diligent in your cleaning of the exposed bone and wound before trying to relocate it back into the skin.

Also, watch that the skin of the wound edge is not trapped by the bone as it returns to its position – use sterilized tweezers in order to prise it clear, if necessary.

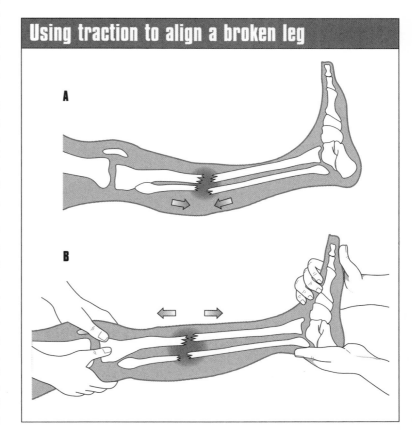

Using traction to align a broken leg

A

B

Bandaging an open wound on the lower leg

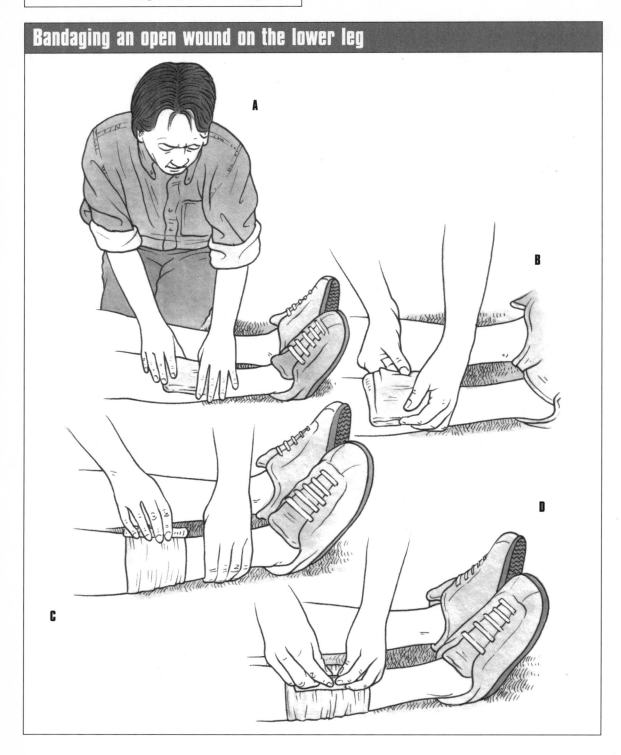

Traction is also applicable for dislocations, and we shall look at specific dislocation injuries shortly. The principle remains effectively the same for dislocations as for fractures, though as you are trying to relocate a joint integration, the process can be more awkward and special techniques required for individual joints. Yet in every application of traction, if the joint really does not want to go in, then do not force it. In these situations stabilize in the injured position as comfortably as possible, keep checking the circulation in the affected limb, deliver pain medication if necessary, and allow the professionals to sort it out.

Once any dislocation or fracture is realigned, your second priority is to stabilize the injured area through bandaging or splinting. Bandaging will be covered when we

look at specific injuries, but splinting is a technique which generally follows the same principles for each situation. Professional splinting materials can be bought from any good outdoor pursuit shop, but perfectly workable splints can be manufactured on the spot in a survival situation.

To make a splint, you will need three main materials. The first is a rigid stabilizer, something like a ski, ice-axe handle, or straight branch, but even flexible materials such as towels, magazines, and coats can be rolled up and used as stabilizers. Secondly, you require binding materials to tie the stabilizer securely to the broken limb – dressing bandages and duct tape are good. Thirdly, you will need some kind of material padding to keep the break comfortable and fixed in place.

Splinting an arm and leg

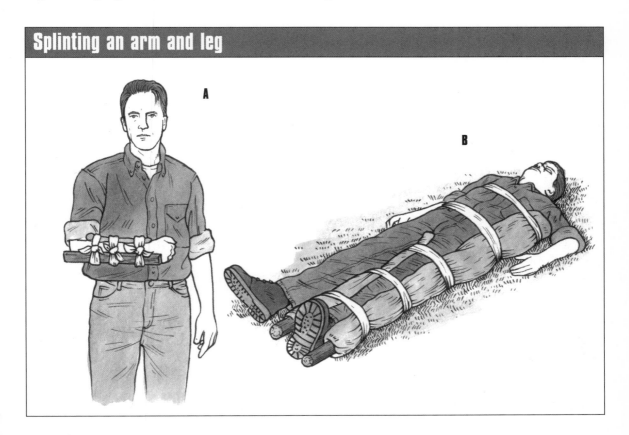

A

B

Bandaging a closed fracture

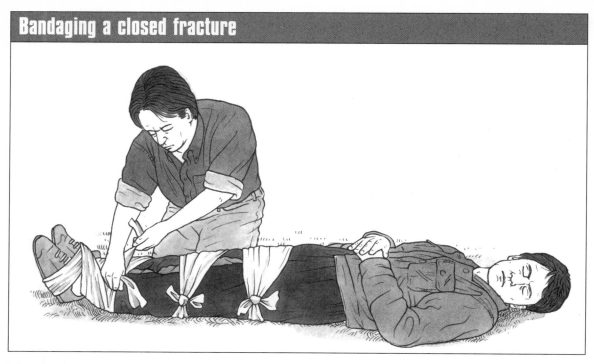

Signs of a broken limb

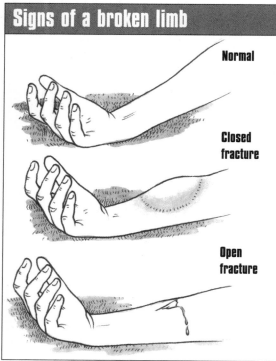

Normal

Closed
fracture

Open
fracture

Actual splinting techniques vary with each wound, but there is a general procedure to follow:

● Only splint a limb which has been aligned or, in the case of a joint, set to the midrange position.

● Bind the stabilizers (or stabilizers, one on either side if required) to the broken limb so that the joints either side of the break are immobilized. For example, if the forearm is broken, the splint should also hold the elbow and the wrist. This is done by running a padded stabilizer down the length of the limb and tying it in place with the bandages. Be careful with the tying so that you are not restricting circulation, so check the colour of the skin and nails in the extremities for signs of infarction.

● If necessary for added stability, bind the splinted limb to an uninjured part of the body. Thus a splinted right leg could be tied to the left leg, or a broken arm tied to the torso. When doing this, however, make sure that there is plentiful padding in between the two body parts.

Once the fractured or dislocated limb is aligned and securely stabilized, then the casualty is ready for evacuation. Maintain a close vigilance over the circulatory situation in the damaged area, and also watch for signs of any localized or systemic infection developing.

For stable fractures that may be the treatment can be modified, as often the casualty will still have use of the limb with pain being possibly the only complication. Splint and support the broken limb, but also use cold compresses to bring down swelling. Then, if possible, elevate the fracture site. In the case of a stable fracture, once the wound is stabilized then if you have the tools and natural materials around you, then it is possible to make improvised crutches to give the casualty some level of mobility (see illustration for building instructions). However, make sure that you know what you are doing with these as badly made crutches can lead to the casualty re-injuring himself if they break or bend suddenly.

Facial fractures

Facial fractures can occur anywhere, but tend to be around the nose, cheek, jaw, or orbit of the eye. Your major concern should be to make sure that the casualty's airway is open and respiration is clear. This is because broken facial bones may alter the dimensions of nasal passages, and also because extensive bleeding might create a fluid impairment of the airway (for serious head injuries see Chapter Five)

For injuries to such features as the cheek and nose, a cold compress should be used to reduce swelling. Cold compresses are made by either packing a cloth with ice or snow or soaking a cloth in cold water. This is then applied firmly to the wound to reduce swelling. The compress will quickly warm when in contact with the skin, so regularly re-soak to maintain coldness.

If the jaw is broken, then the fracture should be supported, but not bandaged, using a soft cloth held just beneath the jawline. Broken jaws often result in a great deal of bleeding and dribbling, so encourage the casualty to lean forward to allow natural drainage away from the airway.

Fractured collarbone

The collarbones act as struts to support the shoulders, and reach from the shoulder blades to the breastbone. Realignment of a broken collarbone is not an option because of its location, so instead the fracture should be stabilized by bandaging.

Place the arm of the injured side across the chest so that the fingertips are touching the opposite shoulder. Then apply what is known as an elevation sling by taking a large triangular bandage from the uninjured shoulder diagonally down under the elbow of the bent arm, and then back up again across the back to tie up at the starting point. Where the bandage supports the elbow, twist up and pin the material so that the elbow is resting snugly in a contoured pocket of material. Then place a pad of material between the bandaged arm and the torso to give extra stability

Dislocated shoulder

A dislocated shoulder occurs when the ball-and-socket joint of the arm bone and the shoulder socket become displaced. This occurs usually after a fall or wrenching injury. Signs of distortion and pain in the area should indicate the injury, as well as a 'flattening' of the shoulder's general appearance. Dislocation will also result in a loss of mobility in the respective limb, and circulatory restrictions resulting from this injury can be acute.

Improvised crutches

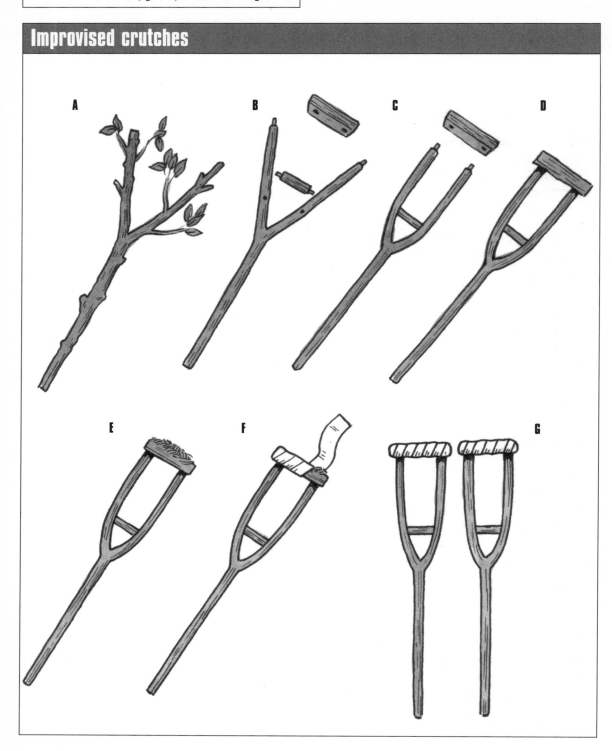

A   B   C   D

E   F   G

Bandaging for a dislocated shoulder

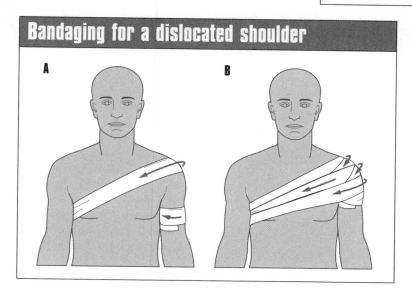

A

B

Traction techniques for relocating a dislocated shoulder can be tricky, mainly because of the muscular strength in the upper body

A particularly effective technique is as follows. Lie the casualty down on a patch of ground, and gently apply traction to the injured arm, pulling with one arm gripping above the elbow. Maintaining the traction, bring the casualty's arm up to about a 90 degree angle from their body, bend at the elbow and rotate the arm

Applying downward traction to a dislocated shoulder

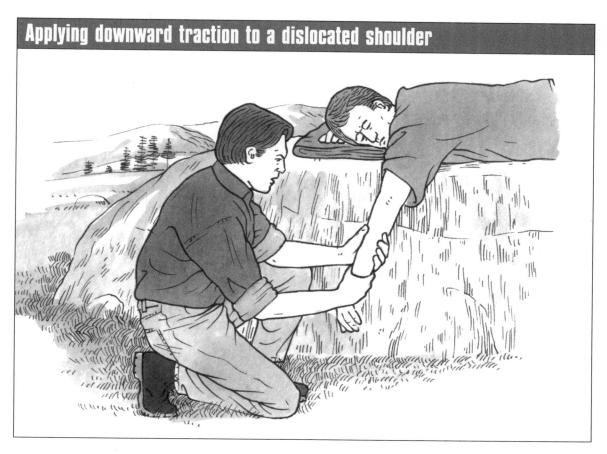

Support sling for a dislocated shoulder

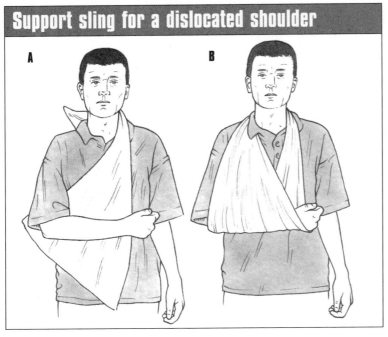

upwards until the final position is akin like someone holding a ball ready for throwing. Hold this position and the traction for up to 10 minutes while the muscles in the shoulder slowly relax. This in itself will usually allow the joint to slip back into place, but if not then watch for a specific moment of relaxation and rotate the arm steadily forward, as if the hand was now 'throwing the ball'. This should relocate the joint.

Another method of relocation that can be successful is to have the casualty lay face down on an elevated

Support sling for a broken elbow

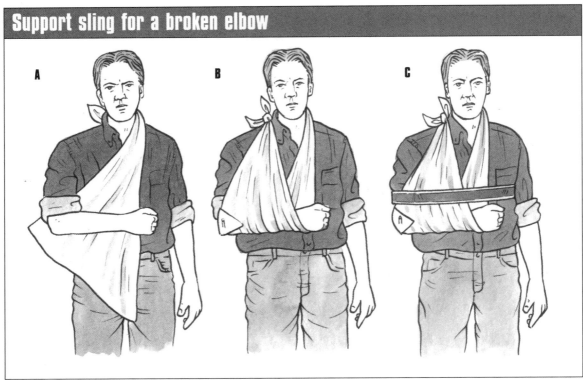

Splinting a broken wrist

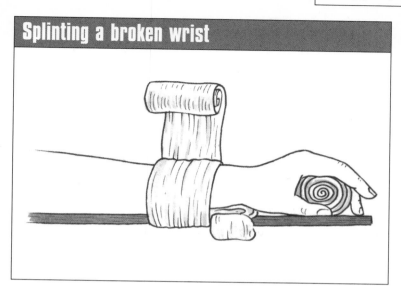

an unstable one, but if it appears to be a stable injury, a simple arm sling will suffice to keep it in place and secure.

An injury to and around the elbow is slightly more complicated. A break just above the elbow will be indicated by the usual signs of breakage, but also by a general immobility in the joint, particularly if the head of the radius bone is damaged in any way. If the elbow is in a bent position, then put in a standard arm sling or splint in this position (known as the mid-range position, when there is roughly a 90 degree bend). If it is in the stretched-out position, then simply put padding between the arm and the torso, and

surface with the arm of the injured shoulder hanging over the side. Take hold of the dangling arm, and maintain downward traction for about 15 to 20 minutes. Once you gently let go, the shoulder should relocate itself. Use whichever of these two techniques most suits the situation.

Once the joint is relocated, then the arm on the injured side should be stabilized in an arm sling. This can be done by taking a large piece of material from the uninjured shoulder, wrapping it underneath the arm with the material supporting from the fingertips to past the elbow joint, then tying the loose ends behind the neck or across the chest. Then shape the bandage around the elbow joint as described in the section 'Fractured collarbone' above, and place padding between the arm and the chest.

Fractured arm and elbow

The arm can be fractured in several different locations. These comprise the humerus (the arm bone above the elbow), the elbow itself, the two bones which comprise the forearm (the ulna and radius), and the wrist. For fractures to the main arm bones and wrists, treat them as for any fracture. Splint if the injury is

Finger dislocation

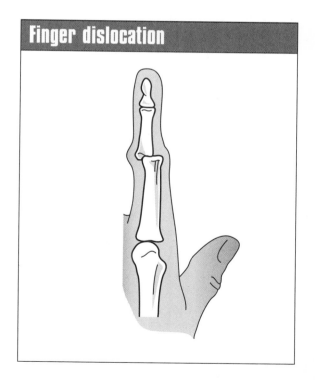

then tie the arm to the torso (wrapping the bandages right around the body) at about three different points to support the entire arm's length. Do not tie anything directly over the wound itself.

Fractures and dislocations in hands and fingers

Dislocated fingers are some of the most common injuries suffered by outdoor enthusiasts, particularly amongst new climbers and

skiers. The dislocation occurs when the force of something striking or pulling on the fingers lifts one or several of the fingers out of joint, and which often happens during falls when the hand is used to break the impact.

Finger or thumb relocation is straightforward enough, though it can take some work. Grip the dislocated section of finger in one hand and the other section in the other hand. Apply firm traction, initially in the direction the finger is pointing in before

Support sling for fractured collarbone

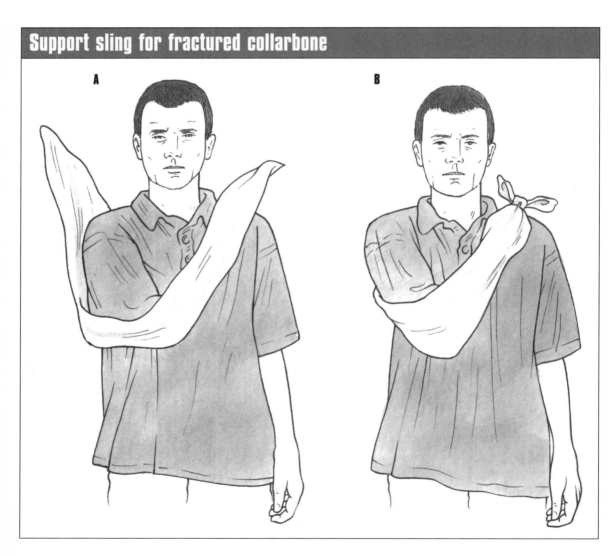

A

B

moving it back into a natural line and slipping it into position. Then splint the finger in the mid-range position.

If the hand has suffered broken bones or fingers, the best treatment is a protective one. Remove rings and watches prior to the development of any swelling, and wrap the hand in soft material. Then place the arm in an elevation sling to counteract inflammation. If necessary, you should splint the individual fingers using pens or pencils as stabilizers.

Fractured ribs

Fractured ribs can cause serious respiratory distress, and dealing with complications and associated injuries such as chest puncture wounds are covered in Chapters Three and Four.

The general symptoms of uncomplicated fractured ribs are severe chest pain – especially when breathing in – as well as concomitant bruising and swelling on the chest wall.

Once you have dealt with any major wounds, sit the casualty up with their body angled towards the injured side. The arm on the injured side should be placed in an elevation sling. But beware while conducting this manoeuvre – a life-threatening complication can occur when a broken rib punctures the lung resulting in tension pneumothorax. Observe chest movement as the casualty breathes (does one side move more than the other?) and look out for signs of distress.

When diagnosing fractured ribs, listen to the casualty's account of his own status. If the pain is not too severe and respiration is not affected, then the ribs could simply be cracked. The casualty should be evacuated in these circumstances, but the problem is a non-serious one and even a hospital will probably dispense little more than painkillers. However, always err on the side of caution.

Bandaging broken ribs

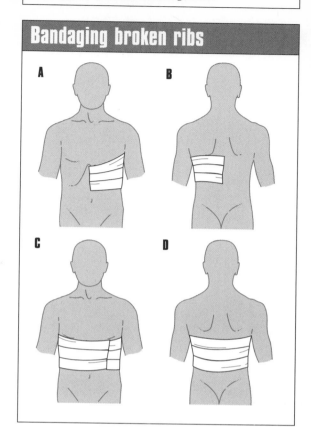

Fractured pelvis

A broken pelvis is a serious injury because it can threaten to damage major blood vessels and the internal organs of the lower abdomen. Pelvic damage is most likely to have been suffered by those who have had a serious fall, taken a tumble in a ski accident, or been crushed in something like a car accident, a rock slide, a tree fall, or an avalanche.

Combined with a relevant historical diagnosis, the signs of pelvic fracture are fairly clear. The casualty's lower limb mobility will be extremely painful or impossible, and the casualty may not even be able to stand (check for leg injuries though). Pain will probably wrap itself right around the lower torso, and blood may be leaking from the penis, vagina, or anus, with further evidence of shock.

Immobilizing the leg as broken pelvis treatment

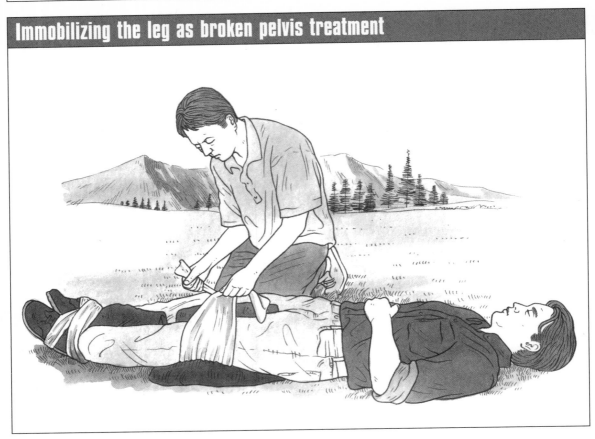

Leg splinting technique

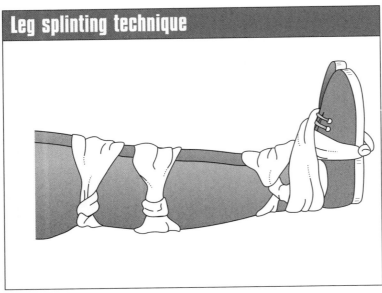

The more severe the symptoms, the more urgent is removal to hospital. Stabilize the pelvic area by placing a padded material between the casualty's legs running down between his knees and ankles, and then binding his legs and feet together securely with bandages (check the toes for circulation), but if this dramatically increases pain then desist. Place a shallow roll of material beneath the knees in order to provide further support, and either rest the casualty or stretcher him out in this position. Treat for shock as you normally would.

Hip, thigh, and lower leg injuries

Fractures to the hip bones (femur) are rare because of the great strength of both the bones and the large amount of powerful muscle surrounding them (though such fractures are more common in the elderly whose bones become brittle through age). Dislocations of the hip are even rarer for this same reason. The treacherous potential of a hip fracture, when it does occur, is that the huge trauma needed to accomplish the injury can often result in bleeding from the major femoral artery (amongst others) – a seriously life-threatening situation.

The symptoms of a fractured thigh are an acute pain in the thigh, loss of mobility, shock, and a compression of the thigh length as the thigh muscles pull the leg shorter in the absence of a solid bone stability. Traction is an immediate measure, and will help reduce blood loss and tissue damage within the thigh.

Pull from the ankle along the line of the limb, preferably while someone else supports the leg at the knee and ensures correct alignment. Once this is done, then splint the casualty's injured leg to the uninjured one in a manner similar to that described for pelvic injury above. The differences are that you should bandage while maintaining traction, and make sure that there is padding between the knees and the ankles. Be careful, however, not to tie a bandage directly over the fracture site – leave this clear. Once the bandaging is done, then you can release the traction. Keep a close watch out for the signs of shock, and evacuate or arrange a rescue immediately.

In the case of a dislocated hip, traction and relocation can be applied in much the same way as the method just described. Yet the power of the thigh muscles may make this a very difficult job; do not persist if the attempt is repeatedly unsuccessful or is producing excessive pain.

If a fracture injury is located in the bones of the lower leg (there are two, the shin bone, or tibia, and the splint bone, or fibula), the treatment follows the same principles for a femoral fracture. Traction should align the leg to its proper position, and the injured and uninjured legs bound together above and below the fracture. With all leg injuries when the two legs are bound together, always remember to tie the knots over the uninjured leg.

Knee injuries

Injuries to the knee can occur in many different ways owing to the complexity of the physical structure. Most vulnerable are the patella, or kneecap, and the ligaments which connect the femur, tibia, and fibula bones, and any violent twisting motion, a blow to the knee or imposing too much pressure of the knee can displace the kneecap, tear or strain the ligaments. The primary symptoms of either of these injuries are joint pain, knee immobility, and a localized swelling of the knee joint.

Dislocated kneecaps can often be relocated, and this should be attempted if there will be a wait of more than two hours for professional help. Have the casualty sit up and then gently try to straighten the leg. The knee cap may pop in of its own accord as you do this, or you can try giving it a guiding push with your thumb. However, if the leg does not want to straighten or the pain is too intense for the casualty, do not attempt to force it. If you have managed to relocate the kneecap, splint the joint for stability. Try not to let the casualty walk on the knee for some time, as this can often result in a re-dislocation.

For injuries to the knee, such as torn ligaments or crushing injuries, then it is best to simply place the knee in the least painful position before stabilizing it with padding around the joint. To bandage the knee, follow

Support bandage for an injured knee

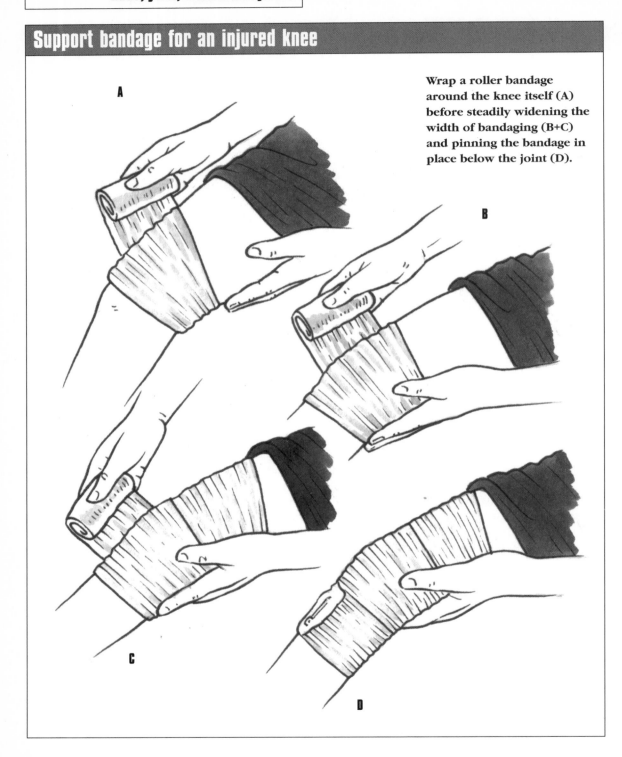

A

Wrap a roller bandage around the knee itself (A) before steadily widening the width of bandaging (B+C) and pinning the bandage in place below the joint (D).

B

C

D

the bandaging technique described in Chapter Four and the illustration in this chapter; make your padding support the entire knee and not just the site of a bleeding.

Fractured foot

The large number of small bones in the foot make techniques such as traction largely irrelevant unless dealing with broken toes, which can be aligned and then bandaged to the healthy toe next to it for stability. Fractures in the foot are awkward in an outdoor setting because they usually result in a serious swelling of the feet, which makes boot wearing impossible.

As soon as a foot fracture is incurred, elevate the foot and then apply a cold compress to the wound site. Then bandage it to provide some measure of stability. It is unlikely that the casualty will be able to walk on the foot for extended periods of time, but if they have to, making a pair of improvised crutches can help (see above).

General points

If you know that rescue is within easy access of the casualty (under two hours), there is no need to perform difficult traction and relocation treatments unless you think that this is important to reduce internal bleeding, such as in a thigh injury. If rescue is expected within a short time, then do not give the casualty anything to eat and drink, as this will make the use of anaesthetic problematic.

SPINAL INJURIES

Spinal injuries warrant a section of their own because their implications can be extremely life-threatening. As explored in Chapter

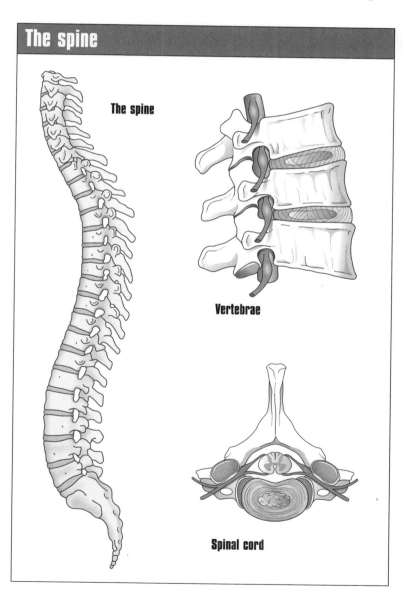

The spine

The spine

Vertebrae

Spinal cord

Stabilizing the neck

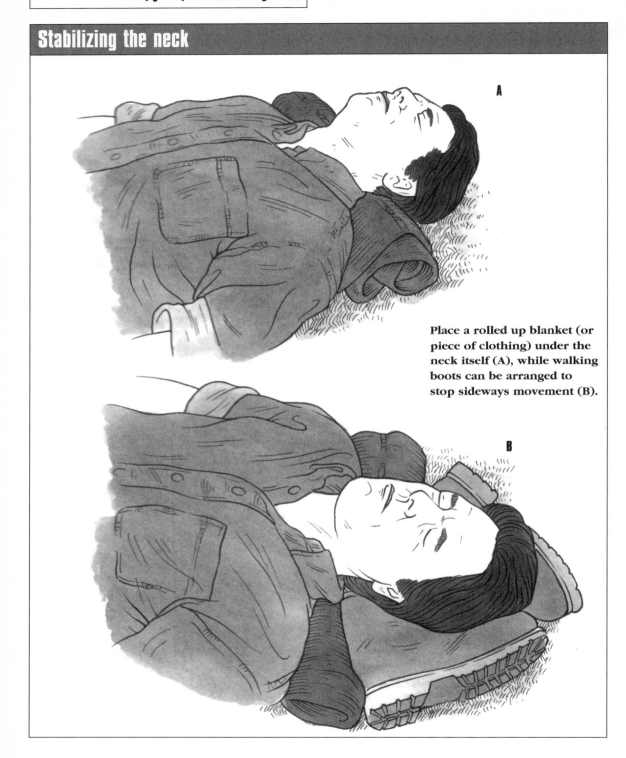

Place a rolled up blanket (or piece of clothing) under the neck itself (A), while walking boots can be arranged to stop sideways movement (B).

Three, the spine contains the spinal cord which is an integral part of the central nervous system. The spine's structure is composed of multiple vertebrae, bones which form a flexible S-shaped stack from the top of the backside to the base of the skull. It is through these vertebrae that the spinal cord runs. Each vertebra is separated by a disc which provides protection for the spine from impact.

Spines are damaged for various reasons. If the casualty has fallen, or experienced a dramatic deceleration such as falling and being restrained by a climbing ropes, or if the casualty has twisted the spine or received a blow to the head, neck, or back, treat him as if his spine is damaged. Caution is warranted. Damage to the spinal cord can range from permanent paralysis and respiratory failure to almost instant death.

Injury assessment

The areas most likely to be injured in a spinal accident are the neck and the exposed bones of the lower back. As a first aider, your initial priority is to check their vital signs, and to ensure that they do not move or that they are not moved by others. Even if they insist that they would like to sit up, do not let them until you have made your diagnosis.

To assess for a spine injury, ask the casualty (if conscious) to inform you of any pains in the neck or back, and also look and feel

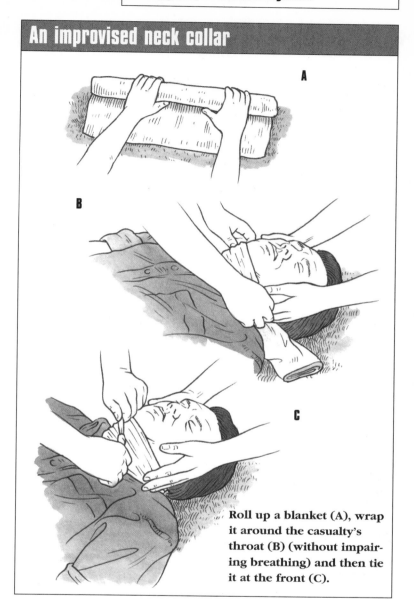

An improvised neck collar

A

B

C

Roll up a blanket (A), wrap it around the casualty's throat (B) (without impairing breathing) and then tie it at the front (C).

along the spine if possible for any signs of irregularity, swelling, or misalignment. Take your assessment further by testing for injury to the spinal cord. This is indicated by tingling, burning, or numbness in the limbs, paralysis, respiratory difficulties, and a lack of response to sensation. Try scratching or pricking the soles of the feet and the palms

Normal spine alignment

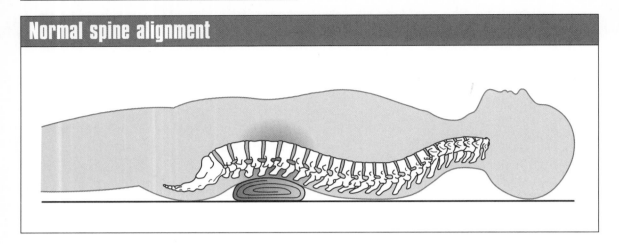

of the hands to see if they twitch through natural response. Also ask the casualty to do the finger squeeze and foot resistance tests (see Chapter Two) to find out if they still have the ability to exercise their muscular control.

Should the casualty not indicate any problems after this diagnosis, then it is more likely that they have suffered straightforward bruising to the back. If, however, they have failed any of the tests, then you should treat as for a spine injury.

Stabilizing the head

Once you have diagnosed spine injury, rescue and evacuation attempts will be put into action immediately. Do not let the casualty move. Instead try to support the head and neck in the correctly aligned position – nose in line with the navel, and the head at its natural angle in relation to the shoulders. If it is not in this position, then grip the head firmly with both hands over the ears, and turn the head into its natural alignment very slowly without jerking or irregular movements.

Once the head is aligned, then you should try to stabilize it with some form of collar. This can be made from something as simple as a towel or magazine. Using a magazine or newspaper, fold it until it is neck width, then wrap it in a piece of cloth with loose mater-

ial hanging over the paper at each end. Bend it over your thigh, and then place this centrally over the front of the throat, pass the loose material around the neck (without moving the neck), cross it over, and then tie at the front. Check that the airway is not in anyway constricted. If you do not have the means to make a brace, then simply place packs and material supports at either side of the head to stop it from moving to either side.

The process of treating a spinal injury so far described assumes a conscious casualty. However, if the casualty is unconscious – which is a very bad sign in someone with a spinal injury – then you should observe the above stabilization procedure, but also be rigorous in your checks of the vital signs and repeat them every five minutes. If you do have to resuscitate, do not tilt the head too far back during resuscitation, as this can aggravate the injury and put more pressure on the spinal cord.

Ideally, a spinal injury casualty should never be moved. Unfortunately, that ideal sometimes cannot be fulfilled in a survival setting. If you have to get the person onto a stretcher, or roll them over to gain better access for resuscitation, then have as many people as possible, working in tandem – preferably five – supporting the body along its length. Ensure that there is one person

The RICE procedure

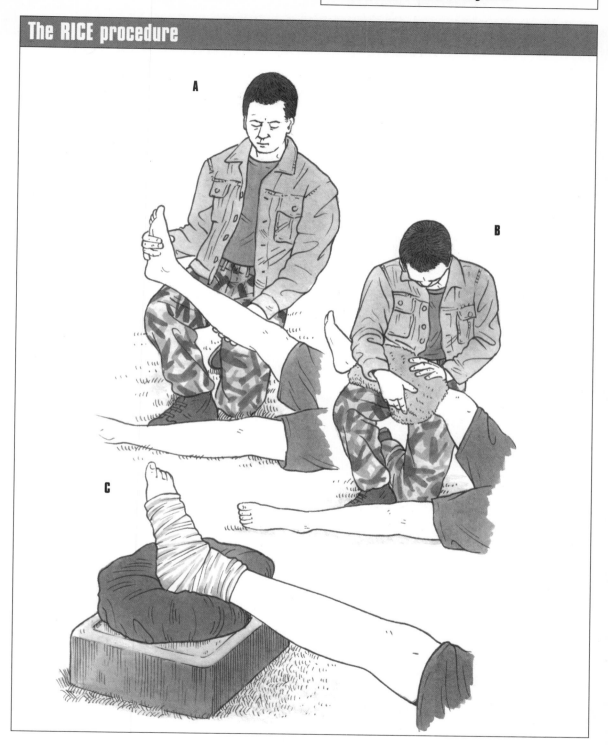

Moving the body into alignment

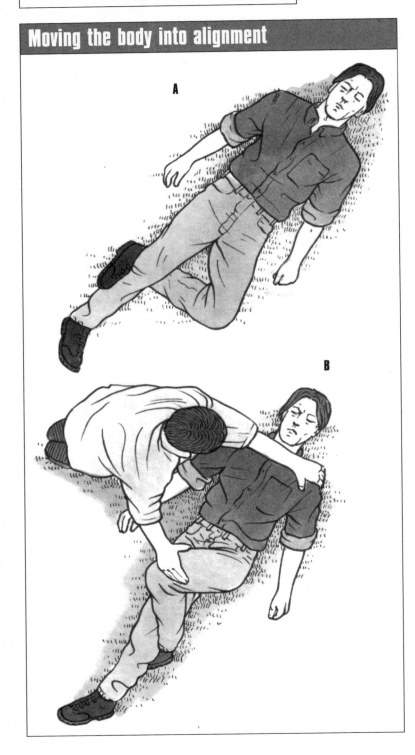

who is dedicated to keeping the head in line with the spine and shoulders.

This will enable you to put the casualty in the recovery position if absolutely necessary. If you do have to move the casualty, make sure that all movements of the people helping to move them are slow, gentle, and controlled.

SPRAINS, STRAINS, AND BRUISES

Sprains, strains, and bruises are the everyday hazard of the enthusiast of outdoor pursuits. However common, they can also be extremely debilitating injuries and if these injuries are incurred in an unforgiving environment, there is the possibility that they will become dangerous.

Though sprains, strains, and bruises can happen to many different parts of the body, there is a usual procedure for treatment. This procedure is also applicable for stable fractures and it is commonly known as the RICE procedure:

- Rest the injured part;
- Ice the injured part – chill the wound with an ice pack or cold compress;
- Compress the injury;
- Elevate the injured part.

This four-stage procedure can dramatically reduce the

swelling which commonly accompanies these types of injuries.

We will illustrate the procedure by referring to a sprained ankle, but the same could be used for any limb or bruised area of the body. Severe bruising on body regions other than the limbs naturally means that elevation is most likely not an option.

Take the casualty's twisted ankle, and immediately elevate, while applying a cold compress directly to the injury for about 10–15 minutes. Then wrap the ankle in a elasticized bandage or some other compressive bandaging – this compression will also help to reduce swelling. However, check that the compression is not too tight, and release it briefly every hour to aid circulation. Keep the ankle raised in this recovery position.

Give ibuprofen or other anti-inflammatory and painkilling drug as needed and according to the instructions and only if you are qualified to administer such drugs. If necessary, with a bad sprain or strain, the ankle or any other limb can be splinted in order to provide some extra healing support to the affected area.

A slightly more problematic situation is that of inflamed tendons, ligaments, and muscles. This usually happens as a result of overactivity and constant wear and tear. Inflammation is often associated with those activities that involve regular motions such as canoeing, walking, and skiing. Rest is actually what is needed, but of course this is not always possible in the outdoors.

The treatment above is still relevant to this type of injury, though it is the warmth treatments that will provide the most beneficial help unless there is an immediate swelling. Most importantly, try to alter the way in which the casualty does his activity, or the length of time he spends doing it. This will help to give the injured area a rest from the affective movement.

With all the procedures outlined above – but particularly the case of fractures and dislocations – do not try to perform the treatments if you are not sure of what you are doing. Steer well clear of certain treatments which may appear natural, such as massaging a sprained joint, which does little good and may actually encourage inflammation.

As with all first aid procedures, prior training is invaluable for handling these situations successfully, so make the investment before you travel.

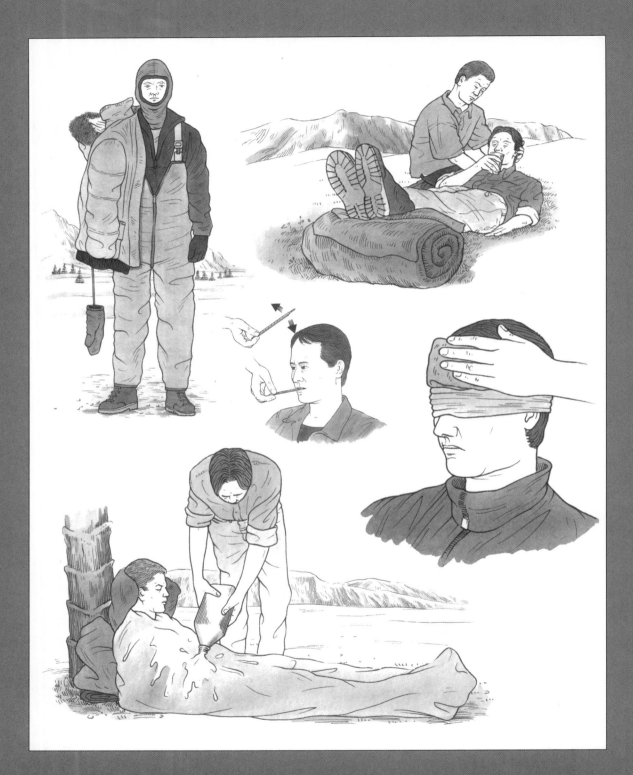

CHAPTER EIGHT

Temperature, climate, & environment

Human beings are highly adaptable creatures. Yet the elements which they face in a survival situation may go beyond the limits of what they can endure. Extremes of heat and cold can overwhelm the body's capacity to regulate its core temperature, and the first aider needs to act fast to restore the natural balance.

One of the many miracles of human physiology is the body's capacity to regulate its own temperature. Regardless of whether an individual is living in a freezing Alaskan hinterland or a tropical rain forest in Brazil, as long as he or she is healthy and appropriately clothed, then the body will maintain its core temperature at 36–38°C (97.8–100.4°F). Yet this temperature control system is vulnerable, and never more so than in outdoor survival situations where the climate and environment can be stacked against anyone trying to stay warm or release heat. This chapter is of special relevance to the outdoors first aider. In it we will review the main threats posed by heat and cold, and specific climate-related ailments such as snow blindness and trench foot.

However, at the outset it must be emphasized that before you travel to any place or country, find out as much detail as possible about the climate. Even the most experienced travellers and soldiers have been caught out. During the Gulf War, a number of SAS soldiers lost their lives to hypothermia while on covert operations – one of the worst blizzards in decades hit the desert region, and the troopers were not appropriately clothed. Their fate was primarily down to bad luck rather than bad judgement, as the weather conditions could not easily be predicted. This is not the case for most of us pursuing outdoor activities.

Wherever you are destined, be exhaustive in your efforts to discover everything you can about the climate that you will face. Do not just look at temperature averages; find out about the climatic extremes that are possible in your destination at the particular time of the year you will be there. Think about temperature, but also consider rainfall, snowfall, humidity, altitude, hours of sunlight and darkness, windspeeds, water temperature, and the possibility of fog. Only when you have this information, purchase or gather the appropriate clothing (see Chapter One). The natural world is incredibly unforgiving at times, so guarantee that you are prepared.

THE MECHANISM OF BODY TEMPERATURE

The human body's ideal core temperature ranges between 36–38°C (97.8–100.4°F). If the core temperature (the temperature within the internal organs and brain) goes above or below this, then problems begin.

Human temperature is regulated by external activities and internal processes. Externally, we generally respond to heat or cold by varying the level of clothing we are wearing, the nature of our food or drink intake, or the posture we adopt. If it is very hot, we will (cultural limits permitting) wear as little clothing as possible, drink cold drinks, sit near fans, and expose our bodies to as much fresh air as possible to maximize heat loss. (Think of the way you hang your limbs over the side of your bed on hot nights to offer as much skin as possible to open-air cooling.) Conversely, on cold days we put on thick layers of clothing to keep our body heat in, move about more to increase muscle activity and thus warming blood flow, take in hot food and drink, seek out sources of warmth, and generally tighten up the posture (for example, sticking hands under armpits, pulling the head down to the chest) to reduce the area of skin open to heat loss.

At the true centre of our temperature control, however, are internal and involuntary processes. Most human heat is generated as a by-product of the conversion of food to energy within human body tissue. Deep within the brain, located within the hypothalamus, is a heat regulation centre which monitors the human body and recognizes if there is the need to conserve heat, or lose it to maintain the core temperature. The processes of these activities are as below:

Heat retention
- Blood vessels in the skin contract to keep warm blood in the centre of the body. Thus our extremities (nose, hands, and feet) are the first parts of our body to become cold in low temperatures.
- Sweating is reduced to prevent heat loss by evaporation on the skin's surface.
- Muscular activity can sometimes be increased through shivering.
- The body's hairs are erected to trap in any heat lost through the skin.

- More of the body's stored fat is burnt up to provide greater energy and heat.

Heat loss

- Blood vessels in the skin dilate, thus transferring more heat to the skin surface where it can radiate its heat away into the atmosphere (which is why people go red in the face on hot days).
- Sweat gland production is increased, with heat being taken out of the body as the sweat evaporates from the skin into the cooler air.
- Breathing is increased to exhale warm air in the lungs, and increase the intake of cool outside air, so assisting the cooling of the blood.

Taken together, the internal and external processes of temperature control are fairly dependable and rugged. Yet sometimes the system cannot cope. If climatic or environmental pressures mean that the body cannot keep its core temperature within the safe limits, then serious and life-threatening conditions can ensue. We now turn to these conditions, their causes, diagnosis, and treatment.

DISORDERS CAUSED BY HEAT

In very hot conditions, the body attempts to cool itself by radiating heat from the surface of the skin and by the evaporation of sweat; hence we sweat more in hot weather.

However, hot climates can present two major challenges to the body system. The first is that once the outside temperature reaches the same level as the body's core temperature, then heat cannot be radiated away (heat exchange can only take place between dissimilar temperature zones). This increases our reliance upon sweat evaporation. An increase in sweating means an increase in fluid loss and hence the possibility of volume shock through perspiration alone, something which can be treated by increasing fluid intake. More serious, however, is when high temperatures are accompanied by high humidity. Saturated air stops the process of sweat evaporation from the skin, and in this situation, the body can no longer control its core temperature which then starts to climb. This can be serious for someone engaged in strenuous outdoor activity such as hiking or climbing, as studies have indicated that sweating levels can actually start to reduce over a period of prolonged exertion.

Once the body system cannot cope with the external temperatures imposed upon it, heat exhaustion and hyperthermia can result.

Heat exhaustion

Heat exhaustion does not necessarily involve a dangerous rise in the body's core temperature, though it is a serious indicator that that process is to come, if left untreated. Heat exhaustion is actually dehydration, this giving rise to volume shock. It is a preventable condition if your party is vigilant about keeping fluid intake high, having regular rest periods (especially if some participants are unfamiliar with the level of activity), and watching out for any of the symptoms of heat exhaustion developing.

The symptoms of heat exhaustion can be as follows. Both pulse and respiration rates are increased, and the skin tone will often be pale and clammy with sweat. The casualty will seem less coherent or responsive in mental attitude, and is easily confused. He could also be experiencing cramps in the arms, legs, and abdomen, owing to the loss of body salt through sweating (this is known as heat cramps, and may be experienced as a separate complaint in hot climates). The casualty's urine output will be reduced as the body attempts to save water. Nausea, vomiting, and a pervasive weakness throughout the body will make the casualty increasingly weak.

Pinch test for dehydration

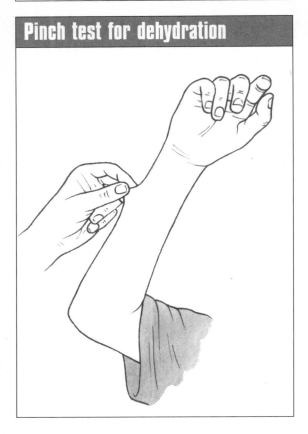

Your essential treatment priority is to get the casualty cool and rehydrated. If an individual loses about one fifth of their body fluid, then they will most likely die of their loss. Particularly serious dehydration is characterized by such symptoms as mental shutdown and delirium, a swollen throat and tongue which disallow swallowing, and shrivelled skin which, when pinched, does not spring quickly back to its original position. Heat exhaustion is the primary stage of this degeneration so act fast.

First, stop the casualty from exercising and place them in a cool and shaded spot. Get them to lie on their back, feet elevated, and give them small, frequent sips of water. Because they have also lost body salt, if possible dissolve about 0.5–1 flat teaspoon of salt (but be careful not to give more than this

as salt initially can make the condition worse) and eight level teaspoons quantity of sugar per litre of water. This should replenish lost salts and sugars, and is also the treatment for heat cramps mentioned earlier.

Keep up this treatment, along with a regular monitoring of vital signs, until the casualty's levels of consciousness and comfort return. Try to wait until the casualty's urine output has returned to normal. Experience of dehydration has demonstrated that this can take a good while, as a dehydrated body can easily soak up several litres of water before surplus fluid is released.

Heat exhaustion is a serious condition. Even if the person seems fully recovered then their evacuation should be put into action.

Hyperthermia (Heatstroke)

Heatstroke, or its direct-sunlight induced equivalent, sunstroke, are life-threatening conditions requiring rapid emergency action. Once the casualty has reached this stage, his internal thermostat has failed, and the result can be coma and death through the damage wrought by overheating. It should also be noted that heatstroke is not only caused by environmental pressures, but can also be brought about by fevers or other illnesses which attack heat regulation.

Heatstroke shares many symptoms with heat exhaustion, but takes them to a more severe level. Pulse and respiration may be racing and the casualty may come in and out of consciousness. Skin could be either pale and clammy (though sweating usually has stopped) or very dry and hot. The most telling symptom will be given by a thermometer reading – their temperature will reach above 40°C (104°F).

Naturally, the most pressing priority here is the rapid cooling of the body. However, be careful. Do not plunge the person into a cold stream, river, or other water source – this sudden chill may actually increase the body's

Treating heat exhaustion

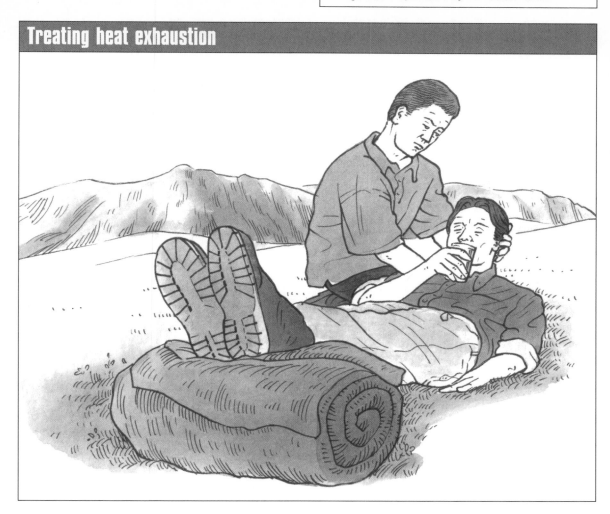

core temperature through shock reaction and worsen matters, or the casualty's body temperature may even reverse and go into hypothermia. Immersion can be done later, and only for short controlled periods, after more appropriate initial cooling.

Initial cooling can be carried out by two methods, in both cases after removing the outer clothing:

- Strip the casualty down to their underclothes, soak or spray them with water, and then fan them to increase evaporation from the skin.

- Cover the casualty with a sheet which you then soak with water. Keep soaking the sheet to keep it cold.

(If the case is very severe and death is likely, once the initial cooling begins to take effect, immersion can be performed. Do this slowly and massage the body continually to keep the circulation pumping out from the core of the body, thus accelerating heat loss. Remove immediately as temperature falls.)

As these techniques are applied, keep diligently checking the vital signs. Especially watch the thermometer reading. Once this drops to close to normal you can stop the cooling, but be vigilant as the temperature may climb once again. Also watch that the temperature does not fall dramatically, and always cover the casualty lightly to ensure that a chill does not set in.

Once the casualty returns to consciousness, perform the same process of rehydration demanded of heat exhaustion above. Keep checking the vital signs, and move them out of any wet clothes and into dry ones. The casualty still needs urgent evacuation at this point. Heatstroke can inflict serious brain damage or other complications, so professional medical control is essential.

Minor heat disorders –
Miliaria

Miliaria is more commonly termed Prickly Heat. This non-serious but irritating condition is caused by the blockage of the body's sweat ducts in very hot weather, usually precipitated by a lack of acclimatization to the weather conditions, the presence of dirt, and the rubbing of clothes. The blocked glands mean that the sweat leaks into the epidermis where it produces two main types of inflammatory disorder (there are more types but are less common).

The first is miliaria crystallina in which the sweat leaks into the very outer layer of

Water blanket treatment for hyperthermia

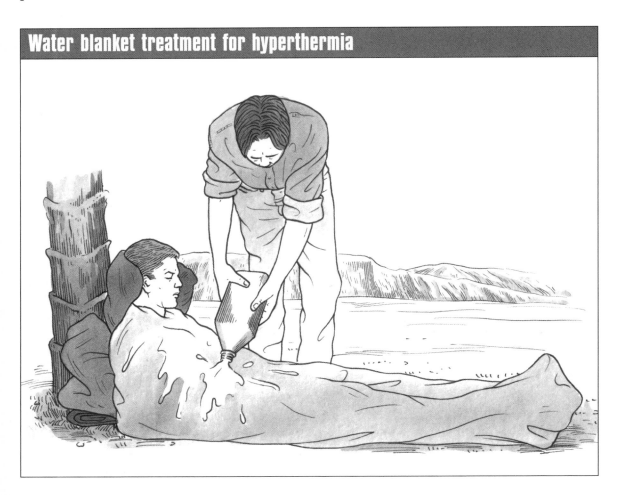

the skin, and produces tiny blisters which give little aggravation (this condition is most commonly seen in sunburn victims). The second is prickly heat proper, or miliaria rubra. This occurs when the sweat leaks into the epidermis and produces inflamed red vesicules, mainly on the torso, arms, and legs, which can become very itchy and irritated. Such a condition is most often encountered in the tropics.

As the sweat pores are blocked, drinking fluids will most likely aggravate rather than heal the situation. Instead, try to give yourself a full body wash and a change into dry clothes, keeping as much of the skin exposed to the air as possible. This should help 'unplug' the glands, and allow sweating to proceed naturally.

Sun glare

The sun's light is intensely powerful, and prolonged exposure in certain parts of the world can make the eyes sore and 'gritty' while impairing vision. Serious exposure can also permanently damage the eyes, effectively cooking the eye. The primary preventative measure against this condition is to invest in a good pair of sunglasses or goggles. You should be prepared to invest in these if you are heading for tropical, mountainous, sea, and desert destinations where sunlight will be clear and strong. The glasses should give full UV protection across the entire spectrum (UVA, B and C) and, if your destination has especially strong sun like an equatorial desert, an infrared filter. This filter can, in effect, stop your eyes being cooked like egg white owing to the sheer heat of the sun. With such eyewear, the dangers of optical damage are negligible.

If, however, someone is suffering from painful eyes and blurring vision, take them to somewhere shaded and wash the eyes with warm water. Then cover the eyes with a dressing, and allow them slowly to recover. Putting dark streaks of charcoal beneath each eye can help limit the glare effect of the sun.

DISORDERS CAUSED BY COLD

Severe cold is just as dangerous as severe heat in a survival situation. Both can jeopardize the body's ability to maintain its vital core temperature, though in the case of cold it does so by extracting heat from the body faster than the body can replace it. When it encounters cold conditions, the body restricts blood flow to the extremities and skin surface, so minimal heat is lost through the skin. This in itself can cause problems, as we shall see in conditions such as frostbite.

However, heat loss can steadily work its way inwards until the body's core temperature is destabilized. Like its opposite, hyperthermia, the condition of hypothermia is one which requires the most incisive first aid actions if it is not to rob the casualty of their life.

For a survivalist, there are a particular range of climatic features which make hypothermia a threat. Low air temperatures are an obvious factor, but often far more important are the presences of wind, snow, rain, or other general humidity. These serve to accelerate the body's heat loss. General rules for the survivalist here are:

- Wear clothing suitable to your environment. That means being waterproof as well as warm, with the ability to change into dry clothes if need be. Keep the hands, feet and head well protected as most heat loss is done through these areas.
- Shelter from the wind if it is taking an unacceptable toll on your body heat.
- Keep moving in a cold climate. Exercise will keep circulation active and supply the body regions with blood flow. This is why you should accept shivering – it is the body's creation of involuntary muscular activity to keep you warm.

147

Cold-weather clothing

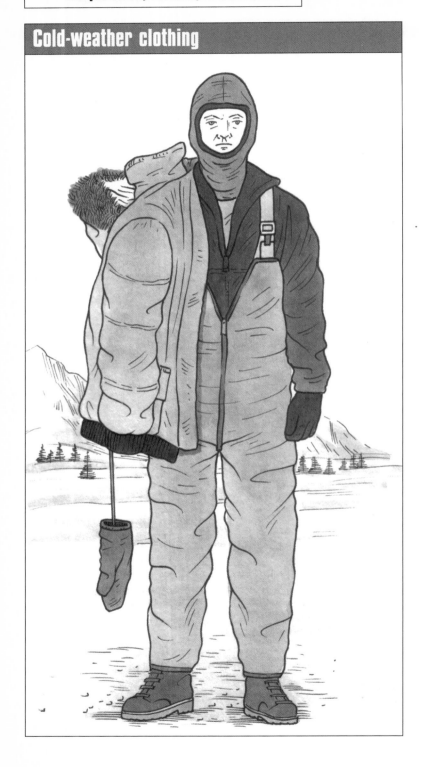

- Make sure that you keep eating and drinking. The body's consumption of calories is dramatically heightened in cold climates, so have adequate supplies of sugary snacks and more complex carbohydrate foods to give both quick and sustained energy levels, and to raise your internal temperature through the process of digestion. Drinking plenty of water is important because urination increases when the body is cold.
- Make an external heat source if need be. Before setting out on any cold-weather journey, be sure that you know how to make a fire and sustain it.
- Hypothermia preys on the exhausted, so be careful if you or any members of your party seem to be especially fatigued.

The world's weather can be astonishingly hard, and even the best-dressed and most knowledgeable can fall prey to cold-generated injuries, especially if they have suffered another injury which inhibits their capacity to keep warm.

Hypothermia
Hypothermia is the condition in which the body's core temperature drops below 35°C (95°F). It is usually caused by excessive

exposure to cold, wet, and windy weather conditions, or from immersion in cold water. The problem with its diagnosis, except in extreme situations such as when the casualty has been submerged in icy waters, is its stealth. Hypothermia can build up over hours as well as suddenly in minutes. A person with mild hypothermia will probably have perfectly normal blood pressure, pulse, and respiration. Yet there are still clear indications which should give cause for concern. Mentally, the person may suffer from sudden, dramatic swings of mood and energy level, lack of concentration, and a tendency to withdraw. Physically they may look pale, with bouts of intense shivering, and their hands and legs may become less agile as the body draws blood away from the surface to the major organs.

At this point, take the person's temperature. This should preferably be done rectally, as the cooling of the extremities may lead to an inaccurate reading from the mouth or armpit. If the thermometer reads 32–35°C (90–96°F) then you should immediately start to treat for mild hypothermia:

- Place the casualty in a position sheltered from wind and rain.
- Make sure that they are warm and dry – change their wet clothing if possible (one item at a time to avoid total body exposure to the elements), and wrap them in a blanket or other protective layer. Non-breathable wraps such as plastic sheets or thermal blankets can stop further evaporative cooling. Also break their contact with the cold ground by placing insulation beneath them.
- Move them next to sources of warmth. This could be a fire or even other people – shared body warmth through hugging will treat them and protect you.
- Get them to eat and drink suitable foods (see above). Do not do this if they are unconscious.

Taking the temperature

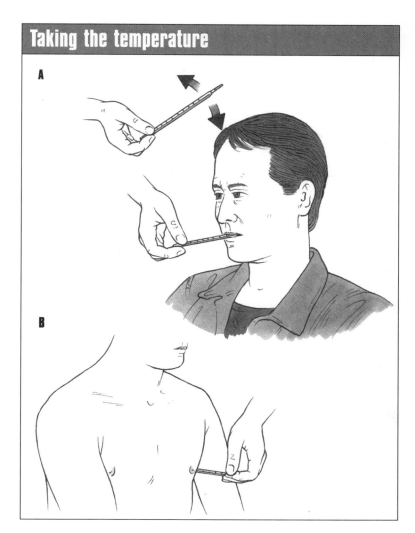

A

B

If all these techniques are applied consistently, then mild hypothermia can be reversed quite successfully, although the casualty should still be evacuated to safety and warmth. Success will be confirmed with the return to a normal temperature level and a better mental state, but keep monitoring all vital signs.

Mild hypothermia, if left untreated or overlooked, can ultimately lead to severe hypothermia. This requires a different level of consideration than mild hypothermia as the symptoms are quite distinct and the urgency is that much greater.

Severe hypothermia occurs when the body's core temperature dips below 33°C (90°F). the symptoms will be much more troubling. Forms of mental derangement may be apparent, and shivering can cease as the body runs out of energy. From there, the casualty can make the steady descent into unconsciousness.

Dealing with unconsciousness

If they do descend into unconsciousness, be careful that you do not misinterpret this as death having occured (although you should also be aware that death is not very far away at this point). Death is easily read, as both pulse and respiration may be almost entirely undetectable in a hypothermic casualty, and their complexion will be icy and cold. To be on the safe side in this situation, start the warming process, and establish if you get any response from the vital signs.

Wrap the patient in warming layers (or alternatively place them in a good sleeping bag), and also a waterproof layer such as a tent ground sheet, in order to prevent any further evaporation cooling. Then apply direct warming using whatever is to hand , such as thermal packs, water bottles, and heated and wrapped stones. Apply these to the armpits and wrists, the back of neck and small of back, the pit of the stomach and between the thighs. These are all places

which have blood supply very near the surface and this blood, when warmed, will travel more directly to the body core. Evacuation is absolutely imperative for a person in this condition. However, move the person with care as their heart muscle is in poor condition. Also keep the casualty flat at all times as this will ensure that the main blood reserves are kept in the core. Be prepared to resuscitate.

Treating for hypothermia

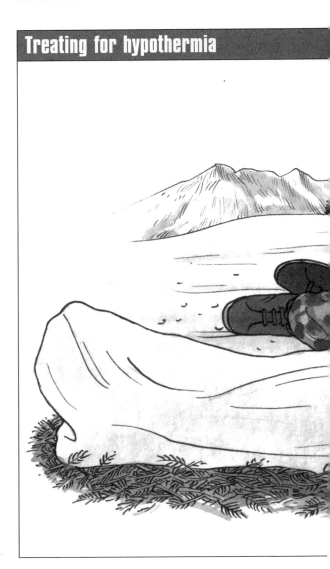

Severe hypothermia is a very serious predicament for the casualty, and survival chances can be slim. Do not give up trying however, particularly if your patient has been recovered after a long time in freezing water.

In fact, the shock of water-induced hypothermia can send the person's body into a kind of suspension, in which the body actually demands less and less oxygen, and so can be revived, even after all vital signs are gone.

Frostbite

Frostbite is defined literally as the freezing of skin and tissue in sub-zero temperatures. It generally attacks the extremities of the body which are most often deprived of blood flow in cold weather. These are the feet and toes, the hands, and most areas of the face, in particular the nose and ears. In all except the most severe weather conditions, and unless a person is suffering from hypothermia,

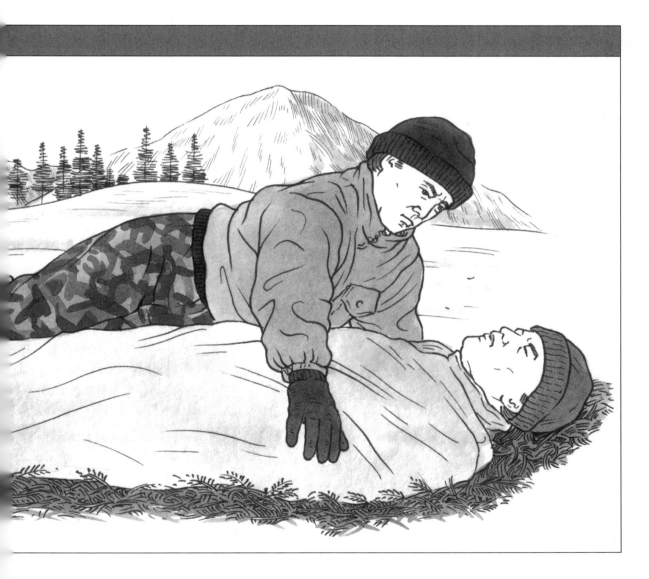

frostbite is generally preventable. Good thermal socks (covered by appropriate boots of course), gloves, hat, and face mask will usually give all the protection you need from frostbite. Be especially careful about leaving part of your body exposed to sub-zero winds, something which applies to skiers in particular who might deliberately cast off clothing on the slopes in their exhilaration, and so might not notice the numbness afflicting, say, their ears, which is an early stage of frostbite. Also do not smoke in such conditions – it limits your physical ability – and keep moving all parts of your body, including your face through different facial contortions. As a first aider, you should watch out for fatigued members of your party who might start neglecting some of their anti-frostbite procedures.

Frostbite is to be taken extremely seriously in all of its stages. If frostbite reaches the advanced stage, great tissue damage can be done by the expansion of the water crystals in the skin. This is even more possible if there is subsequent thawing and refreezing. The damage of the tissue also leads to gangrene. Gangrene occurs when the tissue area literally dies. Eventually the tissue area becomes detached from the body or worse, starts to pump infection around the body which can result in death from blood poisoning.

Degrees of frostbite

The first degree of frostbite is known as frostnip, a thoroughly treatable condition which is nonetheless a forecast of possible frostbite. Frostnip results when there is a freezing in the skin's outermost layers. The symptoms are first pins and needles in the affected area, followed by a change to numbness. The skin colour will be white or grey (pink in dark-skinned people) and somewhat waxy, very cold to the touch. The secret to reverting this condition is simple rewarming. Place hands, for instance, in warm spots such as the armpits or groin, or in the case of other extremities someone else may have to apply body heat or another heat source in the best way available. When the skin becomes slightly red and swollen, with the casualty feeling some pain and discomfort, then the treatment is successful. Keep an eye on someone who has been treated for frostnip, as those areas of the body affected are more prone to refreezing.

If the freezing goes beyond frostnip, the symptoms become steadily more alarming, and more sensitivity of treatment is required.

As frostbite advances, the skin will become hard and rigid, patches of tough swelling appear which can then blister, the colours of the skin go from pale to a variegated blue, and then finally black as the tissue is frozen solid and infected. In these final

Temperature extremes – heat

PLACE	CONTINENT/REGION	HIGHEST TEMPERATURE
Al-Aziziyah, Libya	Africa	57.7°C (136°F)
Death Valley, California	North America	56.7°C (134.5°F)
Tirat Zevi, Israel	Asia	53.9°C (129°F)
Cloncurry, Queensland	Australia	53.1°C (127.5°F)
Seville, Spain	Europe	50°C (122°F)
Rivadavia, Argentina	South America	48.9°C (120°F)
Luzon, Philippines	Pacific islands	40.5°C (105°F)

stages, the frostbitten area will feel exactly like a piece of meat taken from a freezer, and the casualty will find it impossible to move (do not try to manipulate any frozen area – think what happens if you bend a frozen sausage). An ultimate development is when the blackened, blistered areas fall off as dead tissue.

Treatment for frostbite

A primary treatment for frostbite is to make sure that the person as a whole is warm and well clothed; get the person to eat and drink to maintain warmth levels from energy production. Remove any articles of clothing or jewellery which may be restricting blood flow to the area. For the frostbite itself, the best treatment would be delivered in the controlled conditions of a hospital. This is because infection can all too easily occur in insanitary outdoor conditions, and there is still the risk of refreezing, which would greatly compound the damage. Thus, if rescue is possible in a few hours, simply cover and protect the site with a dry gauze bandage and wait for the professionals. If this is not going to be possible for some time owing to the situation, then steady rewarming the casualty is the priority. This involves immersing the affected part of the body in warm water – elbow hot but not uncomfortably hot (about 28°C (108°F) – and keeping it there while adding enough hot water to

keep the temperature constant. The goal is to rewarm the frozen tissue. Always be careful about overheating, and if the casualty's pain starts to become especially severe, this may indicate an over-rapid rewarming.

Once re-arming is achieved, prohibit the casualty's further use of the affected part and cover it lightly with a bandage. Splinting and elevating physical areas such as frozen hands is also recommended as the rewarmed tissue is extremely fragile. Ibuprofen tablets taken according to dosage are an excellent anti-inflammatory. These are useful in stopping blood clots forming in the tissue, and also for controlling the pain which results from a rewarmed frostbitten area or digit. Two things never to do to a frostbitten area: 1) Never rub the area; and 2) never burst any blisters that form.

Frostbite is a difficult condition to treat when outdoors; generally prioritize rescue over treatment when the condition is advanced.

Trench foot

Trench foot, properly known as immersion foot, is an inflammatory condition of the feet (though hands can also be affected), termed after the problem reached epidemic proportions in the appalling conditions of the trenches on the Western front in World War I. It is caused by extended exposure of the feet

Temperature extremes – cold

PLACE	CONTINENT/REGION	HIGHEST TEMPERATURE
Vostok	Antarctica	-89.2°C (-128.6°F)
Oymyakon, Russia	Asia	-67.7°C (-89.9°F)
Snag, Yukon	North America	-62.8°C (-81°F)
Ust-Shchuger, Russia	Europe	-55°C (-67°F)
Colonia, Argentina	South America	-33°C (-27°F)
Ifrane, Morroco	Africa	-23.9°C (-11°F)

to cold, damp weather conditions or persistent immersion in cold water without the chance to dry out or recover. The result is damage to the skin, nerves, and muscles in the affected area. In a sense it functions like a form of frostbite equivalent to non-freezing temperatures, but it can generate serious health problems. Those most likely to be affected are climbers, walkers, and sailors in wet conditions. Tight fitting boots should be avoided, and on any outdoor pursuit a good routine of foot checking and sock changing should be established to catch any symptoms in their infancy. Beware also if you are wearing waterproof boots, as these can seal in sweat dampness and precipitate the condition without contact with the elements.

These symptoms include general inflammation and redness in the affected area, with blistering, infection, and loss of mobility resulting as the condition develops.

The treatment is in effect the same for mild frostbite. Bring the foot naturally back up to body warmth (do not apply any rubbing or water-based heating methods), and sustain it through keeping the feet in dry footwear. Also allow the feet adequate time to rest.

If the condition is advanced, do not burst any blisters that may have appeared. Keep a close watch for any signs of infection (discoloration, pus-seeping wounds) and be prepared to evacuate the casualty if necessary.

Treatment for snow blindness

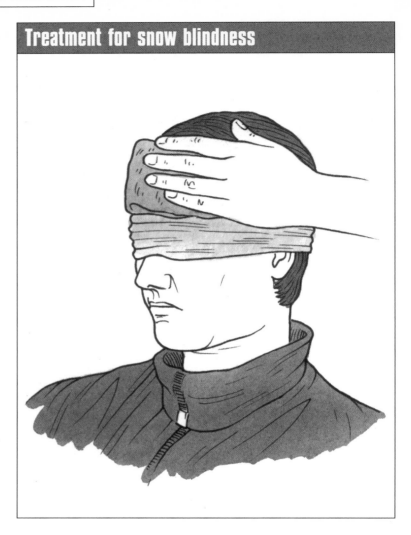

Snow blindness

Snow blindness is in effect the same as the damage caused by sun glare, and can be equally prevented by investment in a good pair of snowgoggles along the same lines as your sunglasses (see above). It is caused by the prolonged exposure to the brilliance of the sun's rays when reflecting off snow or ice. This actually causes a burn on the surface of the eyeball.

The snow-blindness casualty will probably first experience a simple visual discomfort and light aversion, with the eyes squinting and watering, with additional symptoms such as headaches or nausea. As the exposure persists, the eyes will feel gritty and inflamed and vision will become redder or will eventually shut down all together through pain.

The casualty should be taken to a dark place if possible, or have a bandage wrapped loosely around the eyes. The eyes and forehead can be bathed in cold water to bring further relief. If you have any anaesthetic eye drops in your medical kit, now is the time to use them, and you should also give the person use of a pair of sunglasses (or preferably goggles) if there are any available. A makeshift pair of snow goggles can be manufactured by taking a belt, headband, or similar strip of wide material (even cardboard will do), and fitting this over the casualty's eyes with small cross slots cut for eye holes. Smearing charcoal underneath the eyes can also dampen glare.

All illnesses generated by heat or cold are usually preventable in well-organized activities. Always beware of bravado, when members are effectively bullied into continuing to expose themselves to the ailments by the enthusiasm and pride of others for longer than is safe. Though sound first aid practices are listed here, trying to reverse conditions such as hypothermia, heatstroke, and frostbite has no certain outcomes. Should you manage to stabilize the casualty's core temperature, serious physiological and psychological damage can result. Prevention is better than cure.

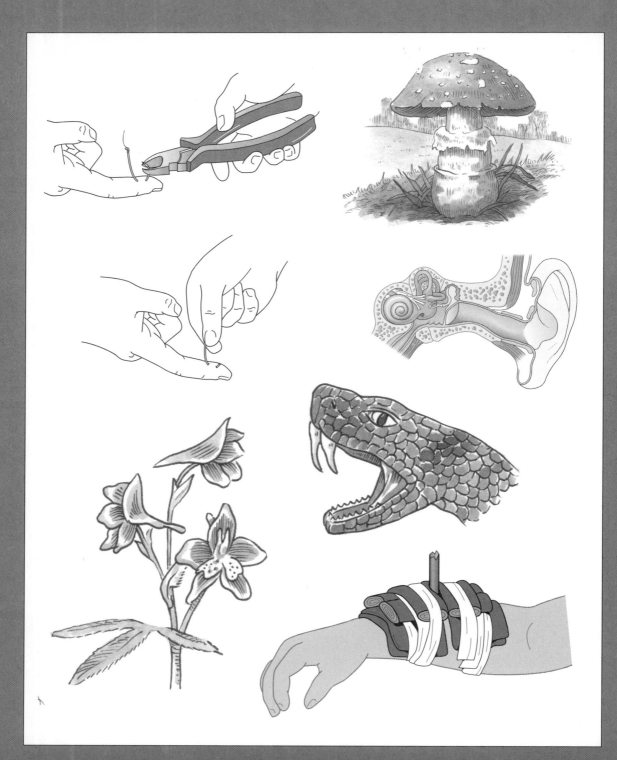

CHAPTER NINE

Poisoning & foreign objects

The outdoor adventurer and explorer is more vulnerable than most to poisoning or invasion from foreign objects, not only from the bewildering array of plants and animals that can deliver powerful poisons, but also from the potentially dangerous tools and equipment carried on outdoor expeditions.

Some general notes on precautions. When travelling to a particular region or country, be diligent in your research about the local flora and fauna. Most will be benign, but in some areas a surprisingly high percentage will not. Find out about everything – from creatures such as big cats which can inflict massive bite injuries, to the invisible parasitic creatures and invasive microscopic parasites that may inhabit rivers. Perhaps, most importantly, if you are going a long way from civilization, know what poi-

sons might be encountered from the natural environment. In some cases, antitoxins related to specific animals can be issued to you in advance of your trip, though many doctors will exercise caution about this as they will not know whether the antitoxin itself might induce anaphylaxis in the casualty.

Once you have assessed the natural dangers of your destination, you should also consider the type of clothing you will be wearing, and the type of equipment you will carry. If you are travelling within a tropical environment, for example, take clothes which will cover you but not cause over-heating. You should also ensure that you pack adequate supplies of insect repellent and insect nets, as well as taking an appropriate antiseptic and antihistamine ointment for treating more common insect bites. Ask your pharmacy or doctor to recommend the most relevant products for your journey to you.

POISONING

Poisons come in a multitude of different guises and can enter the body in a number of ways. Some poisons work on a localized scale, only producing symptoms at the site through which the poison entered. Other, more serious poisons produce systemic effects – they affect the whole body and its vital systems. And yet there are other poisons which will work on both localized and systemic levels.

The most common ways of encountering poisons are:

- **Ingestion** – poisonous materials are taken into the mouth and swallowed. This includes substances such as contaminated food, chemicals, medicines, drugs, and alcohol.
- **Inhalation** – poison is ingressed when breathing in poisonous gases, smoke, or fumes.
- **Injection** – poisons are pushed through the skin from the outside. Typical sources would be snake bite and poisonous plants.
- **Contact** – poisons are absorbed into the skin, typically chemical substances with a high level of reactivity.

Whatever the cause of the poisoning, there are general treatment principles for dealing with most types. The more specific and more unusual cases will be dealt with below.

General poisoning treatments

With every case of poisoning, monitor the casualty's vital signs very closely, and respond as appropriate to problems in respiration, circulation, or nervous function. Also look for localized reactions such as swelling and inflammation, particularly in the airway, and relax any tight clothing or straps around this area. If you find that you have to give mouth-to-mouth resuscitation, then be careful to avoid contact with the source of poisoning.

Poisonous plants and fungi

The outdoor world is abundant with poisonous plants and fungi, and most poisoning from flora sources is through ingestion Do not eat plants or fungi unless you are absolutely sure what they are. If, in extreme cases, you do need to eat unknown plants to survive (this does not apply to fungi), test them thoroughly over a couple of days, first rubbing the plant against your skin on the elbow or wrist, then against your lips, then against your tongue. If there is no reaction after 15 minutes, chew a tiny bit without swallowing and wait 15 minutes more for a response. Again, if there is no allergic reaction, then swallow this piece and wait eight hours for a response. If there is none, then try a very small portion of the plant (about enough to cover the palm of your hand). Again wait eight hours, and if there is no reaction, then it means that the plant is safe to eat (or at least the part of the plant you tested).

Ingestion

Immediately start to monitor the casualty's vital signs. Your most important decision is whether to induce vomiting and thus evacuate the stomach of its poisonous contents. In a domestic setting, you would generally not be encouraged to do this as the professional medical services would be able to make the right diagnosis and give more direct treatments.

Poisonous plants

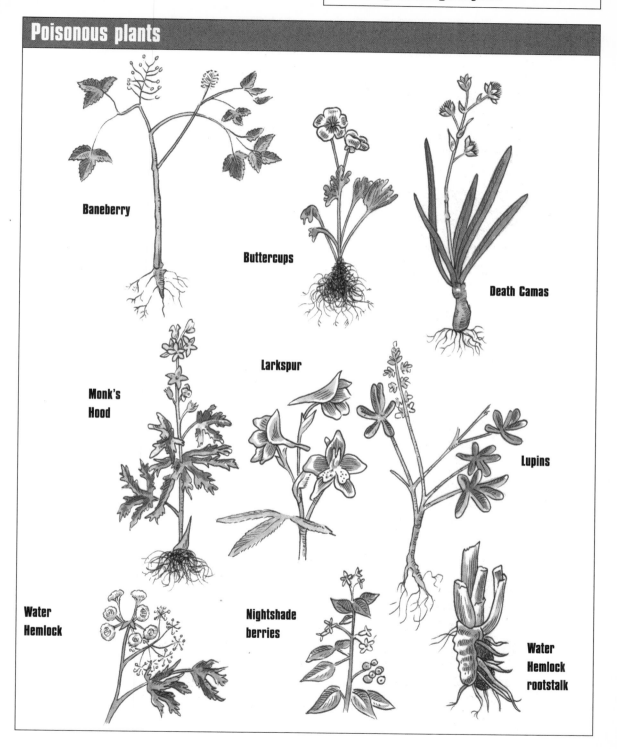

Baneberry

Buttercups

Death Camas

Monk's Hood

Larkspur

Lupins

Water Hemlock

Nightshade berries

Water Hemlock rootstalk

Poisonous fungi

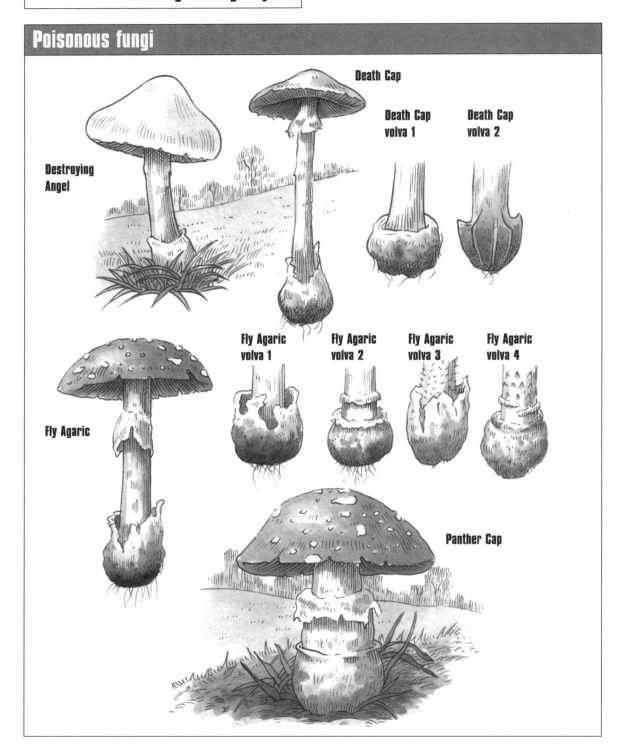

Death Cap

Death Cap
volva 1

Death Cap
volva 2

Destroying
Angel

Fly Agaric
volva 1

Fly Agaric
volva 2

Fly Agaric
volva 3

Fly Agaric
volva 4

Fly Agaric

Panther Cap

However, in the wilderness setting, you often do not have that luxury, so the poison should be brought out of the system as soon as possible. This means immediately upon ingestion and up to several hours afterwards. Note: do not induce vomiting if the poisonous substance swallowed is caustic, corrosive, or petrochemical in nature; this can simply double the impact of these aggressive substances on the windpipe and cause further poisoning. For other plant, food, or medical ingestions, induce vomiting either with a finger down the throat, or with one or two tablespoons of syrup of ipecac and two cups of water. This should bring up the stomach contents after a period of between 15 and 20 minutes.

Once the stomach contents have been vomited, you should then attempt to remove the remaining poisonous content by absorption methods. To does this, give the patient either a mixture of tea, charcoal, and milk of magnesia mixed in equal parts, or just activated charcoal (about 25–50gm [1–2oz]) mixed with water.

These absorption treatments have the effect of absorbing the poison whereupon the charcoal mixture passes out in the faeces as normal.

Contact

In effect, treating a localized skin poisoning is the same as treating a skin wound. The area should be thoroughly irrigated to clean away as much of the poison as possible, and then covered to avoid contact with other irritants. Also ensure that you wash or remove any clothing that may have been in contact with the substance, and which may simply repeat the condition.

A close watch over the casualty should be maintained in case of any allergic reaction with the irritant.

Inhalation

Give the standard form of treatment for problems with respiration (see Chapter Three).

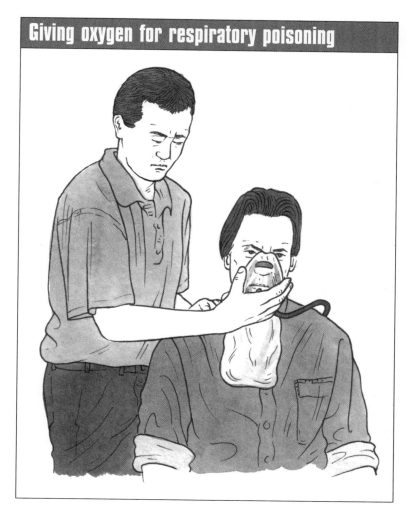

Giving oxygen for respiratory poisoning

INJECTION – ANIMAL POISONS

Animal toxins are some of the most lethal chemicals known to humankind. Their effects are disproportionately varied. A jelly-fish sting, for example, will inject the equivalent to a bad bee sting. However, tread on the spine of an Indo-Pacific Cone shell, and you may find that your life may be at risk. It is impossible here to run through the poisonous qualities of all the deadly or harmful creatures of the world, so we will offer treatments for the generic categories of creatures which you might encounter in outdoor situations.

Remember the old adage that the animals you come across in the wild will be more afraid of you than you are of them. The grounding principle is that if you do meet a snake, scorpion, or other poisonous creature give it space and move away from it in a smooth, calm manner. If swimming in the sea, always wear a snorkel so that you can see what is around you, and ensure that you swim in a pair of sandals or light trainers to protect you from the spines of sea urchins and the like.

Snakes, spiders and scorpions are some of your greatest hazards on land. Some precautionary principles are worth noting. Most accidents with such creatures occur when you inadvertently wander into their habit. Wear a good pair of strong boots at all times, and always check your pack, bedding, and shoes if they have been left unattended for some time, particularly in the morning when the creatures may have used them for overnight shelter. If you are exploring bushes or under rocks, do so using a long stick rather than your hand.

Snakes and poisonous land creatures

All animal bites are dangerous even if no poison is injected because the bacterial presence in teeth makes it very likely that a wound will become seriously infected (some of the most dangerous bites in this regard are those of primates, including humans). However, of a particular concern are the many poisonous land creatures which inhabit the world.

Snakes are probably the most instinctively feared in this regard, and in many

Snake-bite patterns

Non-poisonous

Poisonous

cases quite rightly so. Apart from Europe, which only has the adder to contend with, most other continents have poisonous and lethal species of snake. Snake venom acts differently according to the type of snake. In some cases the only injury will be localized swelling and torn skin, but in many cases there are systemic implications, which will produced results ranging from respiratory arrest to an attack on the central nervous system of the body.

Bite marks

If a person has been bitten by a snake, look at the bite marks as they can sometimes inform you whether the snake was poisonous or not. If there are one or two larger puncture wounds at the front of the bite, distinct from the rest, the chances are that it was poisonous. Do not, however, assume that all bites from poisonous snakes mean that venom has actually been injected. Many times when snakes bite out of fear rather than for food, they do not actually inject. You will know if they have injected any venom, because of the immediate swelling of the wound site, and the deterioration of the casualty's overall condition. However, you should be careful that the last is not exacerbated and is simply hysteria.

Once the casualty has been bitten, regardless of whether symptoms have appeared or not, your main priority above all is evacuation. Try to note the type of snake, or if you are unable to identify it at least note down distinguishing features for the doctors. There is little you can do to negate the effect of the

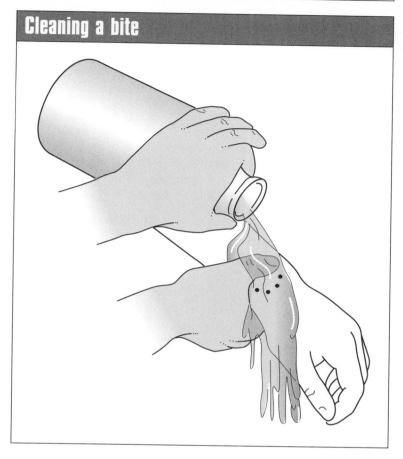

Cleaning a bite

venom itself (unless you have been specifically supplied with antivenoms, and that is unlikely), so keep your priority on basic life support and on slowing the circulation of the poison around the system.

Try to calm the victim as much as possible to slow their heartbeat. Wash the wound site with soap and water to remove any poison which might remain. Then tie a restricting bandage (never a tourniquet) around the bitten limb (if it is the limb that has been bitten) above the bite site; if the casualty has been bitten on the hand, then tie the bandage just above his elbow. This should be tight but ensure that it is not so tight that it restricts blood flow. You can check this by pinching the finger or toe nails. The effect is to restrict the infusion of the venom through the lymphatic system. However, if you find it difficult to control the pressure and you are cutting off circulation, do away with the tourniquet immediately.

In addition to biting snakes, there are also spitting snakes which spray venom over some distances, often directed at the eyes. The effect can be excruciatingly painful, and you should immediately wash out the eyes with water or, if an absolute emergency and there is no water close to hand, you can use urine.

One final point on snakebites. Never try to suck out the poison, it will only endanger you and the casualty even more.

There is a whole range of other poisonous non-flying land creatures, including scorpions, spiders, millipedes, and centipedes and larger creatures such as the Gila Monster and the Bearded Lizard of the Americas. Your treatment principles overall should be the same as that for snake bites. Watch out for any developing anaphylaxis, and give antihistamines according to instructions to reduce the swelling in the localized area. In most cases, a scorpion or spider sting or bite will not be fatal in a healthy adult, even one from such feared creatures as the Black Widow spider.

Aspirin can help to reduce the pain, but the casualty should be evacuated if they become ill from the bite or if the swelling is severe. Time is of the essence, so in this situation, you must move quickly.

Poisonous sea creatures

The sea is home to a large percentage of the world's most toxic creatures, though by their very environment, there is less chance of encountering them unless you are spending a great deal of time in the sea at relevant locations. Poisonous sea creatures deliver their venom in a variety of ways, and with a variety of results. This is principally done by either contact with poisonous spines, such as are found on stingrays and sea urchins, or by nematocysts, the stinging parts of jellyfish, anemones, and octopi amongst other creatures which inject toxins through a multitude of tiny stinging cells, which embed themselves in the skin. Poisonous bites are also encountered in water-dwelling creatures (as well as serious non-poisonous biters), but these are some-

World's most venomous land snakes by region

REGION	SNAKES
Europe	Adder
North and South America	Rattlesnakes
	Copperhead
	Fer de Lance
	Cottonmouth
	Bushmaster
	Coral snake
Africa and Asia	Cobras
	Kraits
	Boomslang
	Mambas
	Russell's Viper
	Puff Adder
	Saw-scaled viper
	Malay Pit Viper
Australasia	Death Adder
	Australian Black Snake
	Taipan
	Tiger Snake
	Australian Brown Snake

what rarer, and tend to be confined to several quite lethal species of sea snake.

As with all toxins, monitor the casualty's vital signs every five minutes or so to check for deterioration. In addition, use the following more localized treatments.

- **Spine toxin** – Clean and tend to the sting site in the manner of a general wound, but be wary of any stinging particles which remain and take these out carefully with tweezers. The wound size will vary tremendously depending on the type of fish or creature encountered – some spines are minute whereas other reach many inches. A distinctive treatment for this type of wound is the application of heat. Place the wound area in hot water, as hot as the casualty can bear, for up to 90 minutes, depending on when the pain retreats.

- **Nematocyst toxin** – Nematocysts remain on the skin to sting and so should be washed off with copious amounts of salt water (not fresh water, which will only encourage further stinging). Once this has been done, scrape the sting site downwards with a solid, flat object (the back of a knife or flat-angled tent peg) then soak with vinegar for about 30 minutes to neutralize the stings. Following this, coat the sting area in a powder (such as talcum) before brushing the talcum off and taking with it the remaining nematocysts.

- **Poisonous bites** – treat as for general wounds and poisoning, but with an added attention to any severe bleeding.

INSECT ATTACK

Insect attacks are possibly the most commonly encountered wildlife dangers for any outdoor adventurer (as I write, my own father is recovering from multiple bee stings through inadvertently treading on a nest). Almost every country which is not in a sub-zero state has its own quota of stinging and biting insects, and in tropical or desert areas the volume of such creatures can reach frightening levels.

Insect attacks can cause a first aid problem for several reasons. Firstly, they tend to cause a significant amount of pain, discomfort, and irritation. Second, they can impart diseases such as malaria (in the case of mosquitoes). Thirdly, they can produce a fatal allergic reaction, either through one sting because of inducing anaphylaxis, or through the toxic overload produced by the many stings of a swarm attack. This usually occurs because the inflammatory reaction to the sting closes up the airway or produces respiratory failure. Fourthly, some insects can induce a significant blood loss during feeding by introducing an anti-clotting agent or a local anaesthetic which ensures that the blood continues to flow until they have stopped feeding.

The treatment of anaphylaxis is treated elsewhere, but your first priority is obviously to remove the sting from the body. This is quite simply done by gripping the sting with tweezers and extracting straight out from the skin. However, you must grip the sting below any poison sac if present, as squeezing the sac will result in the injection of more toxin. With the sting removed, apply a cold compress, or give the casualty something cold to suck if the wound has been incurred in the mouth.

OTHER WILDLIFE PROBLEMS
Ticks

One of the best ways to avoid a problem with ticks is to cover yourself well with your clothing, and avoid showing too much exposed skin, especially in the grassy, wooded environments which are their natural habitat. This is much easier said than done, particularly in very warm climates, so always have a regime of checking your body for ticks as their presence is largely inconspicuous.

Ticks feed on blood by biting into the skin, whereupon their jaws lock very firmly. The problem is not the bite but rather the possibility of the tick imparting disease or infection. Even if a tick is successfully removed, the casualty should be monitored for any developing illnesses or problematic inflammation/rashes at the bite site or on the body in general (these may take some days to develop if infection is present).

To remove a tick, grip it very close to the skin with tweezers – your aim is to grip the head itself. Lever the tick out with a rocking motion. This will hopefully remove the head, but if parts are left behind, try to scrape them out with a sharp knife. Then wash and cover the wound.

Leeches

Leeches are another blood-feeding creature. Long and worm-like, they tend to live in moist, humid, and wet conditions and thus are especially prominent in the tropics. They tend to attach themselves unnoticed by sliding off vegetation and connecting themselves to the victim where they will feed and swell considerably in size. Unlike ticks, they cannot be pulled off, and the best methods of removal are by touching it with fire (such as a lit cigarette or smouldering piece of wood), or by sprinkling the creature with salt. These techniques should make the creature shrivel and drop off. Following this, clean the wound.

Internal parasites

Many areas of the world offer considerable hazards in the form of worms and intestinal parasites which actually inhabit the casualty's internal organs. Access to the casualty is through several routes, though usually through contact with infected water or by a faeces-to-mouth route in situations of very poor hygiene. Inspecting a person's faeces, as unpalatable as that sounds, can actually reveal the worms and so help you to make a firm diagnosis, though some worms are too small to be detected in this way. Hygiene is the key to preventing these diseases. Keep food protected, wash hands diligently before eating, and be careful of where you swim. Once worms have penetrated internally they can be irritating and alarming (some grow up metres in length in the gut), and if left untended, they can eventually become very dangerous.

Here we will quickly run through the main types and observe symptoms and treatments.

Roundworm

A pink or white worm which grows up to 30cm (12in) in length and is spread through the faeces-to-mouth route. Symptoms of roundworm infestation can include coughing (the young worms travel through the bloodstream to the lungs) with blood being brought up, intestinal discomfort, and even a blockage of the gut. The treatment is essentially drug based, and will usually consist of dosages of Mebendazole or Piperazine (a very common worm medicine). However, mixing about four teaspoons of Papaya milk with equal quantities of sugar and honey water can also help to act as a natural de-wormer.

Hookworm

This short 1cm (0.4in) long parasite is acquired either orally through infected water, or by the creature boring through the skin, most often through bare feet (a good reason to keep them covered). Once inside, they travel via the bloodstream into the lungs, from where they are coughed up, swallowed, and thus begin to cause problems in the stomach and gut (their name comes from the way they attach themselves to the inside of the gut). Hookworms are a serious problem. They can cause general fatigue and more critical illness, such as pneumonia and anaemia. They require professional medical treatment with drugs, so evacuate the person or administer the drugs yourself if you have them. Should the person become anaemic (symptoms of anaemia include very pale skin and fingernails, weakness, and even swollen feet and swollen face), feed them iron-rich foods or give them iron pills.

Threadworm

These 1cm (0.4in) long parasites gather around the anus and cause considerable itching. The resultant scratching allows them to get beneath the casualty's fingernails, from where they are inadvertently transferred to the mouth. Cleanliness, particularly before and after a bowel movement, is vital to both prevention and treatment of threadworm. Keep the hands clean and fingernails cut short. Rubbing vaseline around the anus can help relieve itching. Threadworm really needs drug treatment with Mebendazole or Piperazine, but an effective home remedy is to crush four cloves of garlic into a cup of water and drink this once a day for three weeks (if your outdoor pursuit lasts that long).

Tapeworm

The tapeworm can grow to several metres (yards) in length and usually infects into humans through the eating of poorly cooked meat products. Generally their effect is mild, and can cause stomach pain and upsets while they live in the intestines. They can cause more serious problems if the young tapeworms (pork tape-worms only) make their way to the casualty's brain. Tapeworm infection can often be diagnosed if the flat 1cm (0.4in) long sec-

tions of the tapeworm's body are found in the casualty's underclothes or faeces. They need professional medical treatment, so begin evacuation.

Amoeba

These are not worms but microscopic organisms which can enter humans in their millions through insanitary drinking water. Although far from everyone gets ill from the infestation, they can cause the serious condition called amoebic dysentery. If a person has amoebic dysentery, the primary symptom will be very loose diarrhoea, though this may be interspersed with constipation, which can contain mucus and blood (the latter sometimes in serious quantities). Fatigue will be severe, and dehydration can become dangerous. A fever may sometimes be present, though this more commonly indicates bacterial dysentery.

Like other forms of infestation, professionally administered drug treatment is required unless you are trained to do so, so in the interim keep the casualty hydrated by giving them plenty of fluids and restrict their exertion as much as possible.

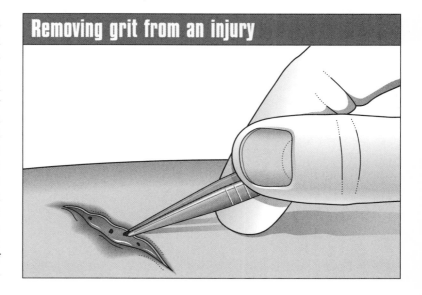

Removing grit from an injury

Bandaging an impaled object

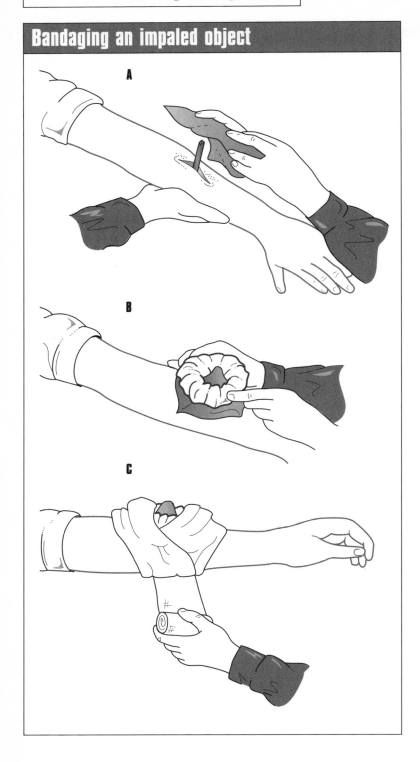

A

B

C

Blood flukes

Blood flukes are a worm which enters the host either through contaminated water or through broken skin. Some flukes can cause bilharzia, a disease of the urinary system which expresses itself in symptoms such as bloody urine or diarrhoea, pain following urination, and a general abdominal pain accompanied by itching and weakness. Drugs such as metrifonate and oxamniquine are the best treatment possible for this condition, so professional help should be found to administer them.

As this run through the world of parasitic invaders implies, there is little you can do in the way of treatment without the administration of appropriate medicines. If your travels will take you to remote parts of the world where such creatures and illnesses are endemic, then you should either take trained medical personnel with you, or be trained yourself in the diagnosis and the treatment of these potentially serious invaders.

FOREIGN OBJECTS

The first aider may not only have to respond to an invasion of the body by outside creatures, but also by intrusion through the skin of various inanimate objects. Climbers and walkers are

Stabilizing an impaled object

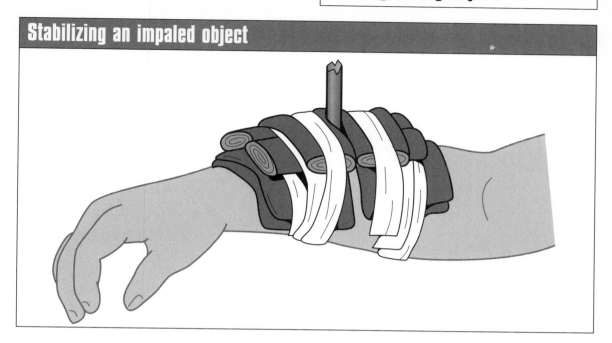

often encumbered with sharp tools and instruments, or surrounded by them in the natural environment (thorns, rock fragments, and so on). We have already examined the process of treating wounds in depth, but now we turn to techniques of handling objects which have penetrated the skin, or affected the eye, the nose, or the throat.

Impaled objects

The treatment for handling impaled objects can be different in a survival and outdoor situation to what would normally be carried out in a domestic or urban setting. If the emergency services are readily accessible, then the correct procedure is to leave the object in place, using pressure techniques to stop the bleeding. The pressure needs to be modified if the impaled object stops direct pressure – instead press hard either side of the wound, pushing the edges of the wound together around the object. Once bleeding is controlled then you should bandage around the object until it is firmly held in place by

the bandages (ideally bandage over the object as well to stop both vertical and horizontal movement). Then you should take the person to professional medical help. This procedure is best as the removal of impaled objects often results in further tissue damage.

If there is little chance of rescue for some time and the casualty needs to be moved, then it is much better to attempt to remove the object yourself, the exception being truly major impalements which go through the torso. To remove an impaled object, do it slowly. Do not keep pulling the object if it is hard set in the wound. If it does move, work it slowly free, stemming bleeding (which may be profuse) while you go. Once the object is clear, then you can dress it as for a normal wound. However, in this situation, you may need to pack the wound with dressing material.

Dramatic impalements, such as those on tent pegs, ice axes, and tree branches, are fairly uncommon. You are much more likely to encounter small objects such as splinters

Removing a splinter

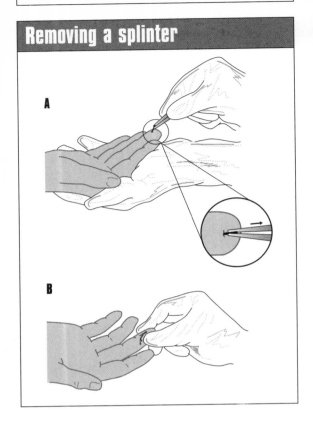

Removing a fish hook

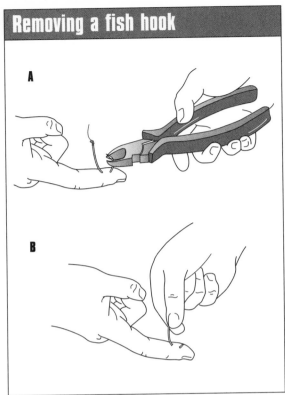

and fish hooks impaled in the skin to a shallow depth.

To remove a splinter, try to grasp it very close to the skin using a pair of sterile tweezers. Ensure that you draw it slowly outwards and against the direction in which it went in.

Once this has been achieved, draw out a little blood from the wound by squeezing it. Following that, you can then dress the wound. If you cannot get the splinter out, leave it alone and bandage it. However, keep checking it each day to see whether or not part of the splinter has presented itself for removal.

Fish hooks, by their very purpose, present a more difficult challenge for extraction. If you have to remove it, cut away the line and, if you have wire-cutters, also the barb. Once the barb is removed, hold the eye of the

The human eye

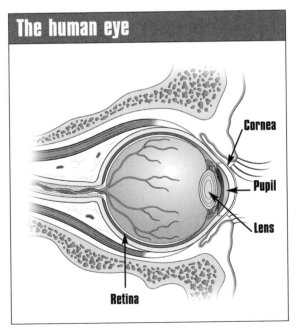

Treating eye damage

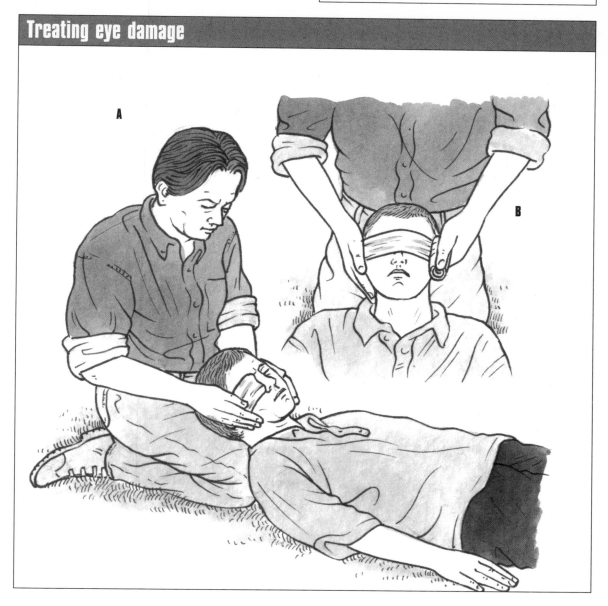

hook and withdraw it, following the shape of the hook. If you do not have wire cutters, or the barb is embedded in the skin, then you will have to push the barb forward and through the skin, then take hold of it with a cloth or other protective material, and withdraw it with the eye coming through last of all.

Drawing out a fish hook can be a very painful procedure for the casualty, so ensure that you do it with a decisive, steady action until it is completed. After that, you can then dress the wound.

Even with small wounds, check them regularly for signs of infection and for signs of general illness. If someone has not had an

Washing out the eye

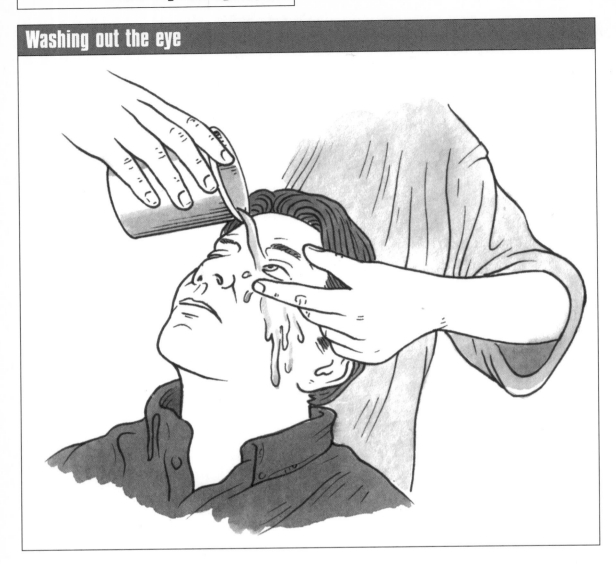

up-to-date tetanus shot, then start evacuation proceedings.

OBJECTS IN THE EYE

Any object in the eye is an excruciating and disorientating injury. If you are in a survival context, as soon as a person is temporarily blinded, then you must immediately act. This is particularly true if they are in a potentially dangerous natural setting, such as when rock climbing.

If a foreign body has entered an eye, immediately prevent the casualty from rubbing it. Inspect the eye yourself by carefully drawing back the eyelids with your finger and thumb. If the casualty can, get them to look in all directions. In this way, they will be presenting all of their eye for your inspection.

Once you can see the object, and if it is not embedded in the eye, then simply try to wash it out. You should irrigate the eye

Removing a foreign body from the eye

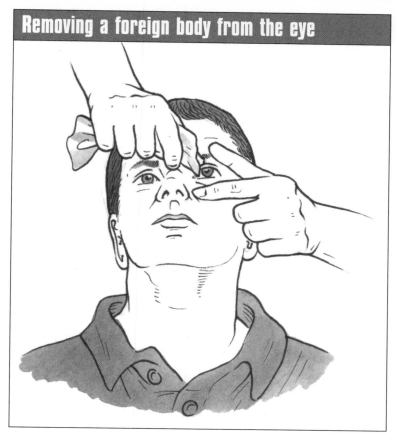

repeatedly with large quantities of water.

Alternatively, if you can clearly see it, you can remove the object by using the edge of a moistened piece of soft, clean cloth which you might have to hand.

One of the biggest dangers with eye injuries is that of infection, a problem that is very real for outdoor people. If the cornea (the transparent covering over the surface of the eye) is cut in any way, the eye may be in danger from infection. Put antibiotic eye ointment if you have it into the damaged eye according to instructions, and then cover the eye with a clean bandage – this can either be taped into place with adhesive plasters, or can be held by a bandage wrapped around the head.

Infection is diagnosed if the eyes appear swollen, reddened, or emit a yellow discharge. If infection has taken place, medical treatment should be sought if it has not cleared up within two days of its initial appearance.

More serious injuries to the eye can result from foreign bodies entering. If there is blood present behind the cornea, or if the foreign object has cut into the eye itself, cover the eye as has been described above, and then immediately start rescue proceedings.

FOREIGN OBJECTS IN THE NOSE

Foreign bodies invading the nasal cavities are quite rare in adults, as their developed reflex actions usually blow out the object on first

The human nose

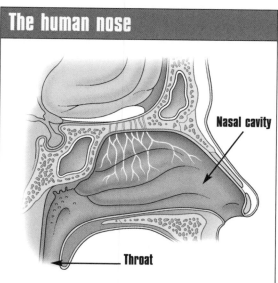

Nasal cavity

Throat

Washing a foreign body from the ear

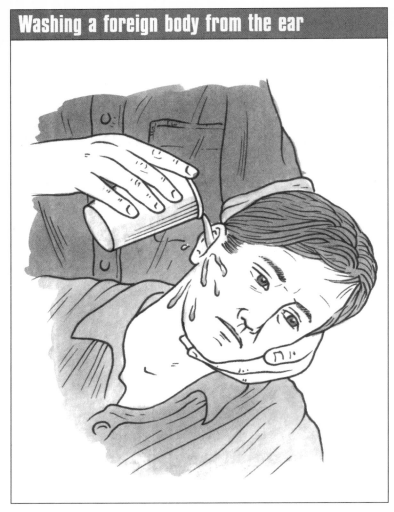

membranes which line the nasal cavity, or worse still, the object can be progressively inhaled until it enters the lungs. Symptoms can include a swollen nose, some difficulty in breathing, or a bloody discharge of mucus.

Unfortunately, unless the object is close enough to the nostrils to be easily extracted, there is little you can do without professional medical assistance. Do not probe deeply into the nostril with an implement, as this may only serve to push the object deeper and deeper into the nasal passages and down towards the windpipe.

Instead, start to evacuate the casualty and maintain a close watch for any signs of sudden respiratory distress caused by the foreign body entering the deeper air passages.

FOREIGN OBJECTS IN THE EAR

Foreign bodies most likely to invade the ear are insects. Ants, spiders, and other creatures can enter the ear when a person is asleep outdoors and close to the ground, as the ear seems to offer the insect possibilities of warmth, shelter, and food (as they often mistake it for another insect hole).

Sometimes, on waking, the casualty is not even aware of the fact that the insect has entered their ear. If a person complains of strange thumping and scratching noises inside their ear, accompanied by woolly hearing and some earache, then insect intrusion

intrusion. This type of accident is actually much more common in very young children, who wilfully put objects into their nose during inquisitive play.

However, the chances of objects intruding into an adult's nasal passages are slightly increased in a wilderness situation because of the presence of insects, which can either fly up the nose or crawl into it when the person is asleep.

Any foreign object up the nose can be potentially serious. Damage can be caused to the delicate blood vessels and mucus

The human ear

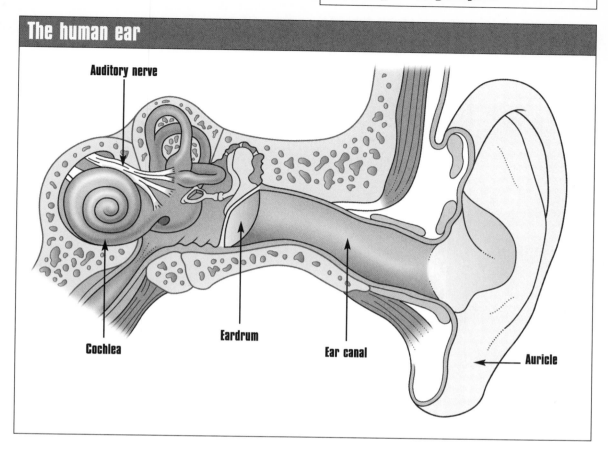

Auditory nerve

Cochlea

Eardrum

Ear canal

Auricle

is a possibility, and should be treated as such (this is, of course, after discounting any other possibilities).

The ear consists of three main parts. Outside the head is the visible, fleshy part of the ear – this is called the auricle. This gives access to the ear canal, which in turn leads down to the eardrum. The eardrum is the membrane which vibrates to generate hearing. These three parts together are known collectively as the outer ear.

Beyond the outer ear is the middle ear, which consists of a small series of bones set in an air cavity through which sound is transferred to the parts of the inner ear. Once into the inner ear, the sound waves are transferred into electrical impulses by the cochlea, and are then sent to the brain down

the auditory nerve for translation into meaningful patterns.

When a foreign body invades the ear, it usually stays in the outer ear. One method of removing it is to literally float it out with water. To do this have the casualty sit or lie down with the problem ear presented flat and uppermost. Then pour a steady stream of warm water into the ear until it floods out, hopefully bringing the insect with it.

Repeat this process a number of times if it does not work initially. However, if floating out the insect with water is still unproductive, start evacuation proceedings. Time is important; if the insect dies in the ear and starts to decompose, then a serious inflammatory infection can result which strikes from the ear into the face.

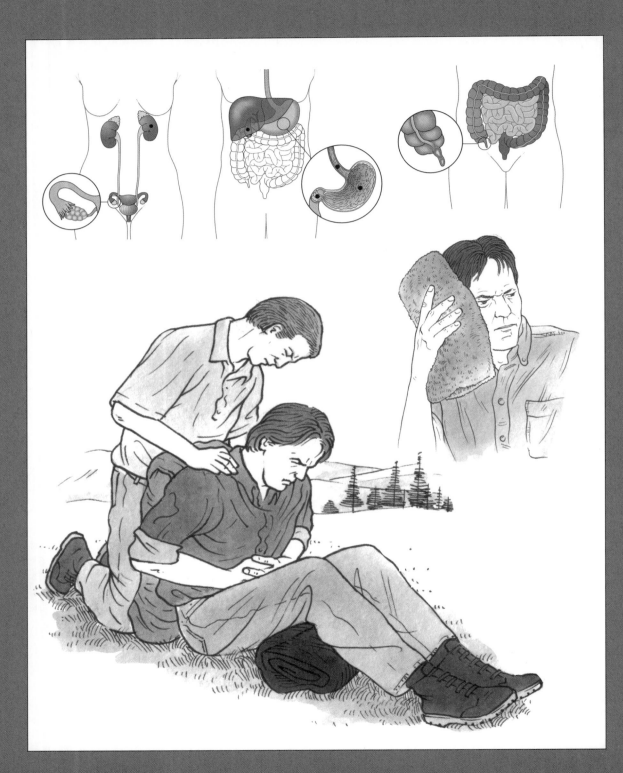

CHAPTER TEN

Other ailments

Most domestic and workplace first aid deals with the immediate treatment of accidents or rapid-effect illnesses such as anaphylaxis. The range of medical challenges encountered by the survival first aider can be substantially broader.

This is principally because there is a wide range of illnesses worldwide which thrive on the unsanitary conditions often encountered outdoors. Furthermore, these illnesses are able to gain a substantial hold as professional medical care is usually far away.

The care of a doctor is exactly what a person needs if he or she falls ill in the wilderness – first aid can only go so far when modern medicines and medical procedures are required. In this chapter, we will run through a broad sweep of miscellaneous complaints, ranging from the serious to the relatively trivial, and provide sound first aid treatments for each. However, in the absence of professional medical staff on your team, you should be aware that rescue or evacuation is usually the end goal of your treatment.

Many of the diseases and illnesses that follow are infectious, so exercise a rigorous hygiene policy around the sick person. If necessary, isolate the casualty from the group, sterilize any utensils used by the patient before they are used by anyone else in the group, and be sure to avoid all contact with the patient's body fluids or waste – even the output produced when the patient coughs. Also be diligent about disposing the patient's body waste well away from your camp, preferably bury it.

APPENDICITIS/PERITONITIS AND ABDOMINAL PROBLEMS

Your appendix is attached to the lower intestine below, and to the right of, your navel. It serves no significant purpose in the body, but if it becomes infected, then the consequences can be serious. Once infected, it swells, causing great pain and illness, and can eventually burst and cause peritonitis – infection of the peritoneum, the membranous sack which contains the human organs. This is a life-threatening situation.

The symptoms of appendicitis begin with a general abdominal pain focused around the navel, but which becomes increasingly severe and extends downwards to the lower right side. The pain may be accompanied by fever, vomiting, and constipation. Further diagnosis can be made by using the rebound test. Position your fingers a little way above the

The appendix

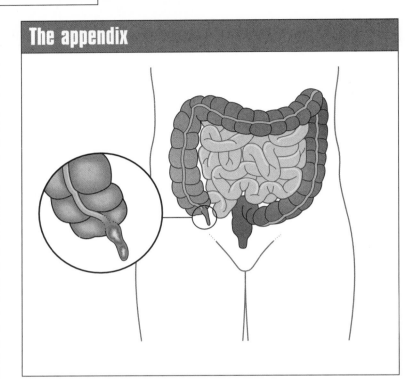

Locating an abdominal complaint

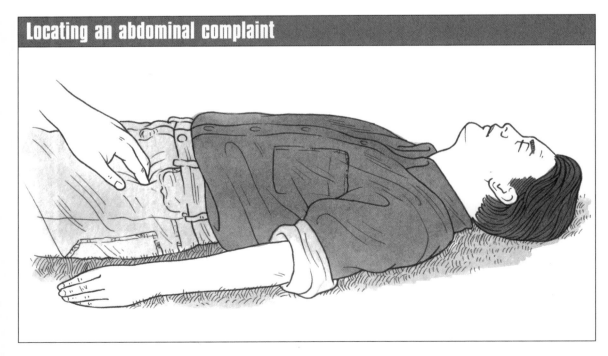

left groin and press down. When the casualty reports that this is beginning to hurt, quickly remove your hand. If a harsh pain hits the casualty when you remove your hand, then appendicitis or peritonitis are the likely causes. If peritonitis is the case, the severity of the illness will increase and the abdomen will become rock hard and very painful to touch.

In either case, surgery will be necessary, so evacuate (using a stretcher) or quickly arrange a rescue. Your first treatment will largely be preventative – do not let the person ingest food or drink, but if dehydration becomes a problem then administer sips of water.

Appendicitis and peritonitis are only two of the wide range of abdominal problems, and it would be impossible to look at them all here. However, with any abdominal pain, if the symptoms include fever, delirium, dehydrating illnesses, or any sign of internal bleeding, then follow the procedure just outlined.

CHOLERA

Cholera is a gastro-intestinal infection caused by ingesting water infected with the vibrio cholerae bacterium. Cholera occurs wherever there are unsanitary conditions, and travellers to any developing countries must have a cholera vaccine in advance.

Treating earache with a warm compress

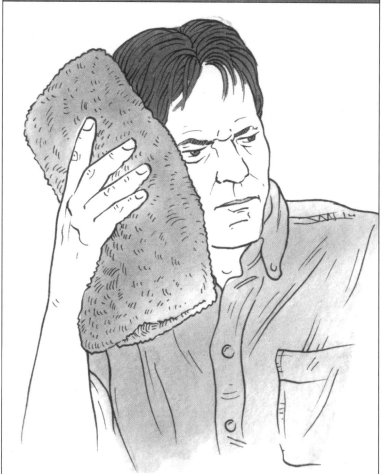

Earache is very common. Causes include an infection in the middle ear, dental problems, a foreign body within the ear, and changes in air pressure. Unless the pain is accompanied by bleeding, discharge, fever, head injury, or deafness, then earache is non-serious. Give painkillers (read the packet) and apply a warm compress (a towel wrapped around a hot object).

Those who die of cholera, as many do worldwide, usually die of chronic dehydration through violent and prolonged diarrhoea. The fluid loss is dramatic. Other symptoms include low blood pressure, muscle pain, fever, and shock. Cholera requires hospitalization as soon as possible, but in the meantime, all you can do is give the generic treatment for dehydration (see below), but with the drinks given almost constantly. One of the problems the survival first aider must deal with is disposing of the waste produced by the cholera patient. If possible, try to improvise some form of latrine over which the casualty can be positioned.

DIARRHOEA

It is often very difficult to pin down the causes of diarrhoea. Food poisoning, change in climate, infection, and overeating can all cause diarrhoea, but in most cases, the complaint will clear up in a few hours, or at most a couple of days. If the diarrhoea persists and the condition is acute, dehydration becomes a serious threat. To counter dehydration,

focus on rehydrating the casualty with half a teaspoon of salt and eight teaspoons of sugar mixed into a litre of water. Administer the water in frequent sips, but do not give any food for 24 hours. After this period, give nutritious food (nothing greasy, spicy, or alcoholic, and avoid raw fruit initially). Soups and broths are the ideal introductory foods, then proceed onto cooked vegetables and plain well-cooked meats.

HAEMORRHOIDS (PILES)

A haemorrhoid results from a clot or mass building up in a vein around the rim of the anus. This swells outward to create small external lumps which can bleed, sometimes profusely enough to warrant surgery. Haemorrhoids are caused in several different ways, most commonly by anal infections or through abdominal pressure such as that experienced when lifting heavy objects, or

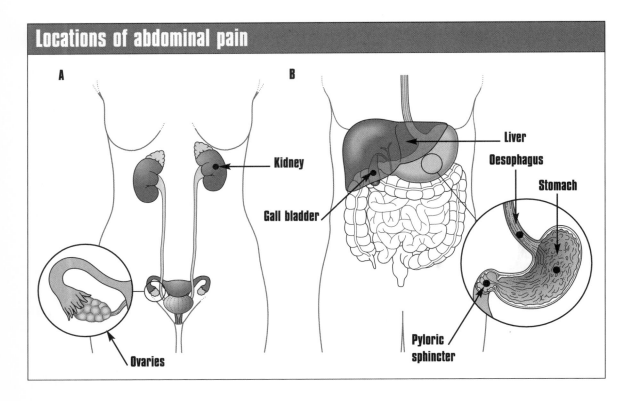

Locations of abdominal pain

A   B

Kidney

Gall bladder

Liver

Oesophagus

Stomach

Pyloric sphincter

Ovaries

Supporting someone with a hernia

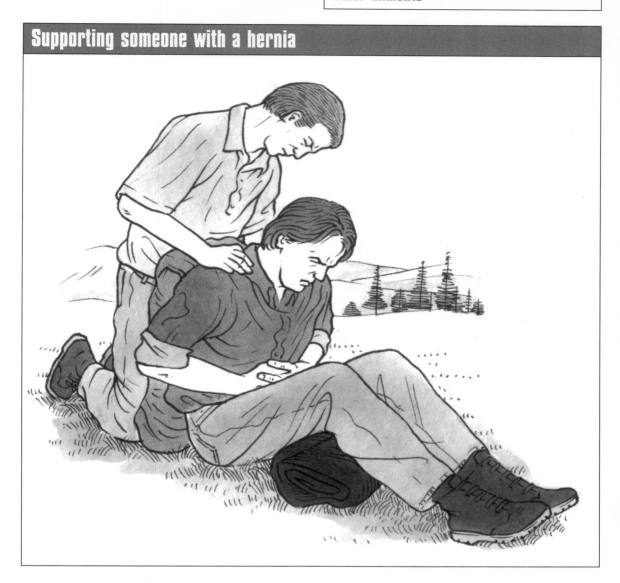

with constipation. Outdoor adventurers can be vulnerable to piles because of the level of exertion on the body. For those who are aware of their condition, suppositories and medications are available. In a wilderness situation, the best treatment is to bathe the anus with warm water (preferably immerse the backside), and eat lots of fruit and fibrous foods to make stools looser and easier to pass. If a pile is bleeding, treat it like any

other wound and apply direct pressure – take it seriously as the bleeding is directly from a vein.

HEPATITIS

Hepatitis is an inflammation of the liver stemming from a variety of causes, and can be both infectious and non-infectious. It is usually transferred when the body waste of an infected person is passed into water or food, which is then ingested by another person. Sexual intercourse is also a primary route of infection. The main symptoms of hepatitis are lack of appetite, abdominal pain, vomiting, very dark urine, and whitish stools, and a yellow tinge to skin and eyes several days after infection.

As hepatitis is a virus, even antibiotics will not help. In fact many medicines will simply damage the liver further. The casualty needs as much rest as possible, so camp down in one spot and bring rescuers in, rather than attempt to walk the casualty out. Give plenty of fluids and encourage ingestion of foods in fluid form, such as soups and fruit juice, which supply nutrients and energy. If the casualty can eat, feed them with fruit, vegetables, starches and proteins, but keep fats to a minimum, as the body will not tolerate them.

HERNIA

A hernia tends to occur suddenly when a person is lifting something heavy or doing a task which requires strenuous exertion. A hernia is actually a rupture of the muscle wall in the abdomen, allowing a piece of intestine to bulge through. This bulge is noticeable and is usually, but not always, in the lower groin. It can be distinguished from the lymph nodes in this region by the fact that it will increase in size if the person lifts anything.

Hernias can be serious because the abdominal muscles may clamp the piece of intestine and actually block the movement of the bowels. This is an urgent situation requiring professional medical care as soon as possible. Symptoms include severe abdominal pain, vomiting (sometimes with faeces in the vomit), and stubborn constipation. If the casualty is suffering from this type of hernia (known as a 'strangulated' hernia, a surgical emergency), place him or her in a comfortable position of their own choosing, and resist giving them anything to drink unless dehydration becomes a problem. Do not give any food at all. However, if the hernia is painless and not creating any inconvenience, there is no cause for alarm. Simply try to stop the person doing any heavy lifting or overexerting themselves.

MALARIA AND DENGUE

Malaria and dengue are diseases spread by mosquitoes, so it is very important to take preventative precautions such as anti-malarial tablets, insect repellents and sleeping nets. It is also easy to confuse the symptoms of the two diseases. Malaria causes feverish attacks that occur initially once a day, but then about once every two or three days. These attacks usually begin with chills and violent shivering, followed by a high fever which can last days, then a period of sweating and temperature subsidence. However, there are other types of malaria which can result in coma and anaemia. Whatever the type, apart from generic treatments for fever (see Chapter Five) the only treatment for malaria is medicinal. If you are travelling to any area known to have malaria then start a course of anti-malarial drugs before travelling, and maintain the course according to directions while you are there. If a member of your party gets malaria, then evacuate.

Dengue is also transmitted by mosquitoes and is also characterized by chills and fevers, though it is often accompanied by a rash which spreads from the extremities across the body. Dengue should cure itself and provide immunity after a few days, though some southeast Asian strains can do more serious damage by inducing bleeding from the skin and internally. Rest and generic treatments for fever, bleeding, and dehydration are the only recourse.

CRAMP

Cramp occurs when chemicals build up in the muscle, often in association with physical exercise when the participant sweats a

Treating cramp in the foot and calf

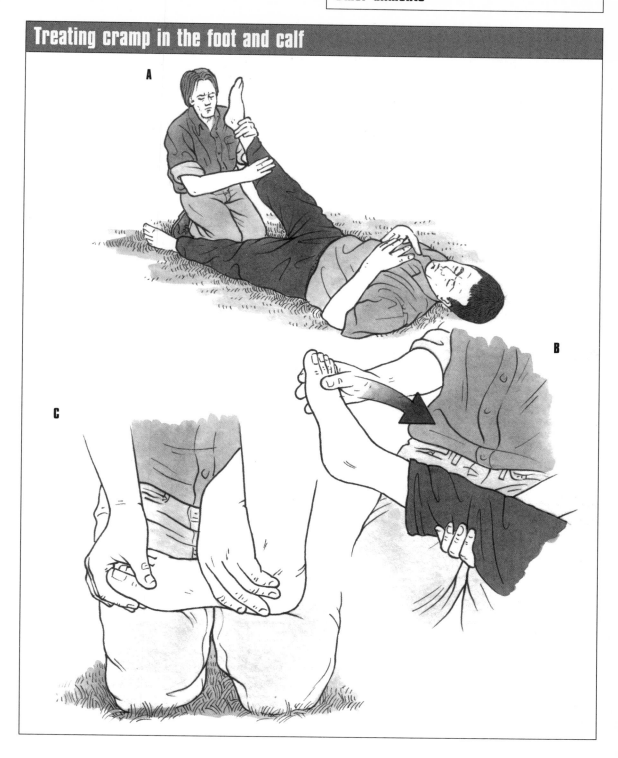

Vaccination which may be required

VACCINATION	NOTES
Poliomyelitis	Areas outside north and western Europe, North America, Australia and New Zealand
Hepatitis A	Applicable to countries with poor sanitation
Typhoid	Applicable to countries with poor sanitation
Yellow Fever	Applies to affected areas; can be compulsory
Anti-malaria tablets	Course taken prior to and during travel

SPECIAL CASES (ON ADVICE OF DOCTOR):

Meningococcal Meningitis	Tick-borne Encephalitis
Rabies	Japanese Encephalitis
Tuberculosis	Diphtheria booster
Hepatitis B	Measles/MMR

great deal. It is a common problem for those on outdoor pursuits, and the strong muscular spasms which cramp induces can disable a limb for many minutes if not treated. Cramp usually affects the legs. For a thigh cramp, elevate the casualty's leg, straighten it if the cramp is on the back of the thigh and bend it the cramp is on the front of the thigh. For cramp in the calf, straighten the knee again and bend the foot back towards the shin, while for foot cramp take the casualty's foot onto your knee, move it back and forth, and massage. Massage should be applied to the affected muscle in all cases, and cramp thus treated should pass away in a couple of minutes.

POLIOMYELITIS

Poliomyelitis is a disease that can cause paralysis by attacking the nerve cells in the spinal cord responsible for motor impulses. It invades orally but not everyone who con-

tracts it becomes ill; sometimes they will just experience a mild fever.

However, when the attack is more serious the symptoms are very much like those of meningitis – severe headache, photophobia (aversion to light), a stiff neck, and vomiting. The casualty either gets better or worsens, developing paralysis in certain parts of the body. Naturally, by this stage, evacuation proceedings should have been instigated by the first aider. There is actually little you can do in the way of treatment. Place hot packs on the muscles to keep them warm. Move the paralysed limbs around to avoid muscular deterioration. Watch carefully for any signs of respiratory distress developing and react accordingly. If the person has to lay in one spot for several days, observe for bed sores – move the person into a different position every few hours to avoid this.

MENINGITIS

Meningitis is a chronic infection of the brain that can easily be fatal. It tends to be confined to children, but can also occur in adults, particularly following another infectious illness.

The symptoms of meningitis are fever and headache, combined with a painful sensitivity to light, a very stiff neck, vomiting, convulsions, and a purple or red rash (the spots do not fade when you press your finger on them). The illness is very serious, and all you can do is to control any temperature imbalances and failures of major systems, while transporting the casualty to professional medical facilities as soon as possible.

RABIES

Rabies is a lethal disease which attacks the central nervous system following infection. The infection itself is transmitted through the bite of an infected animal such as a dog, cat, or bat. A rabid animal can be identified by such traits as foaming at the mouth, an alternately violent, disturbed and lethargic temperament, and death within a week. You may have to kill or cage such an animal if it threatens your camp. If a person has been bitten, clean the bite thoroughly with soap and water, or ideally hydrogen peroxide. Then leave the bite wound open and immediately start evacuation proceedings. It is also useful to try to identify the animal.

The symptoms of rabies in humans are respiratory disturbances, pain in the bite area and throat, problems with swallowing, major personality swings, convulsions, and paralysis (the last symptoms usually precede the casualty's death). These symptoms do not occur immediately but usually develop within two months of the bite, though sometimes they can emerge after a year. Your goal is to move the casualty to a hospital or doctor where they can be given the correct medication before the illness really takes hold.

SWOLLEN FEET

The feet pay a heavy price for activities such as hiking and climbing, and they can often swell considerably through alterations in circulation and over-exertion. To help bring the swelling down, lie or sit the casualty down during rest periods, with the feet higher than the abdomen or head (if lying down), and apply cold compresses. This should help reduce the blood flow to the feet and thus bring down the swelling.

TUBERCULOSIS

Tuberculosis (TB) remains one of the world's biggest causes of premature death, mainly in developing countries (though there is a resurgence of the disease in developed nations). It is particularly concentrated in poor urban areas rather than rural settings, but the first aider should be aware of it due to its extremely contagious nature.

The age group most prone to catching tuberculosis is between 15 and 35. TB is primarily a lung disease though it can actually affect any part of the body such as the neck and abdomen (it can also cause meningitis in children), and can be spread both by respiration and by drinking the milk from cattle with the bovine form of the disease. Symptoms are a severe cough which can contain significant amounts of blood in the later stage, fevers, chest and back pain, weight loss, fatigue, and a hoarse voice.

Someone with TB needs to be taken to a doctor or hospital, and your main role as a first aider is to stop the infection of others. Fashion a face mask which covers your nose and mouth, and wear it when dealing with the person, and keep other members of the group well away (observe them closely for signs of weight loss or coughing). Rest the casualty, and keep them warm and comfortable as much as the conditions allow. Bring rescue to them rather than attempt to walk them out, as they will be very weak.

TYPHOID

Typhoid is an infectious disease passed from faeces to food and water to a human host. Diligent hygiene and appropriate inoculation can make it almost entirely preventable. If it is contracted, it is very serious and requires immediate evacuation or rescue. Typhoid often emerges after natural disasters when sanitation breaks down, and usually comes in epidemics. In such situations, be especially sedulous in purifying water and distinguishing suspect water or food supplies. Mark these as contaminated to warn others. Also set up latrine areas which are distinct from habitation zones.

The symptoms are initially those of a bad cold or flu, but with a rising fever and, distinctively, a slowing pulse (good regular checks on the vital signs are required to spot this). There can also be vomiting and diarrhoea. After a week, other symptoms such as rash, delirium, and weight loss can emerge. Coma and death can be the prognosis if left unchecked.

Your first aid options are limited to general treatment of fever and dehydration until you can get the patient to hospital. Try also to give them nutritional liquids such as fruit juices and soups. One final point is to remember that the casualty can be a typhoid carrier for some time after their recovery, so maintain the separation of their functions.

TYPHUS

Typhus is a similar illness to typhoid in symptoms and result, but it is spread by the bites of infected lice, ticks, and rat fleas. Treatments are as for typhoid, but also make a great effort in your cleanliness regime, washing your body regularly to clean off lice. Also, if you cannot move from a particular area, kill rats with traps and then burn the bodies (do not throw them in waterways as their bodies will contaminate the water which in developing countries may be used for washing and even drinking).

URINARY TRACT INFECTION

Urinary tract infections occur when bacteria are able to multiply in the urinary canal and move up into the bladder (cystitis). As the woman's urethra is a lot shorter than the man's, such infections are much more likely to occur in women. Yet they are also more likely to occur in the context of outdoor adventuring, usually because of unavoidable reductions in sanitation, and also because urination is often decreased through sweating and the germs are not washed out as often. Other causes of urinary tract infection can include (again particularly in women) can include sexual activity and genital trauma or rubbing (such as from a climbing harness).

Urinary tract infections can become serious if they reach the bladder because they can follow through with the spread of infection and cause severe kidney disorders. Symptoms of urinary tract infections can be mild and non-serious. Urination can become painful with a burning sensation accompanying each passage, and it may feel as if the bladder is never truly emptied. More serious is if the infection is followed by a fever, pains in the back and legs (which imply the kidneys are being involved), and genital bleeding. In the serious cases, get the casualty away to the professionals for treatment with antibiotics.

First aid treatments for urinary tract infections primarily involve keeping the casualty's external genitals as clean as possible through regular washing (which they will do themselves), and also making them drink large quantities of water. This increases urination and thus the natural process of flushing out the urinary tract. Taking vitamin C supplements is also a method of treatment as the acidic nature of the vitamin attacks urinary bacteria when the excess which has not been absorbed by the body is passed out.

VAGINAL DISORDERS

The hot, sweaty conditions often produced inside clothing when exercising, and the reduction in opportunities for bathing when on outdoor activities, make women susceptible to vaginal infections and inflammation as well as urinary tract infections. This is usually caused by an imbalance in the levels of 'healthy' bacteria in the vagina which allows yeast to propagate and cause the infection.

The causes of this are multiple, though from the outdoor person's point of view, tight clothing, excessive sweating around the groin, and even psychological state can predispose towards the condition.

Someone suffering from this may have a troubling abdominal pain, a white and thick vaginal discharge, and an accompanying urinary tract infection (see above for treatment of this).

One first aid treatment for this complaint, if you do not have professional preparations with you, is to wash the vagina with a mixture of 1 litre (2 pints) of warm water mixed with six teaspoons of vinegar. If you do not have vinegar, use lemon juice and if you do not have this, use water. Pour the water slowly onto and into the vagina – ideally use a tube which is inserted no more than 7cm (3in) into the vagina. Repeat this process twice a day for up to 14 days. (Never use a douche on someone who is pregnant.)

This may cure the problem, but if it does not then evacuate. If left out of control, vaginitis can result in pelvic inflammatory disorder, an inflammation of the uterus and fallopian tubes which can be serious.

YELLOW FEVER

Yellow fever is a mosquito-borne infection which is present in areas of tropical Africa and South America. It is so called after the jaundiced colour the casualty takes on following infection. This is just one of the symptoms; the others include fever, headache, vomiting (often with a bloody content), constipation, and reduced urination. Treatment for Yellow Fever consists of controlling the fever and dehydration elements of the illness, giving plenty of rest, and allowing the illness to pass naturally, though you should always initiate evacuation as Yellow Fever can leave many complications.

There are many other diseases, infections, and illnesses that can manifest themselves in a survival or wilderness situation, and only a few can be covered here. However, as a first aider, your job is not to cure complex diseases but to get the casualty safely to professional medical care. Always remember this rule. If you do not know what illness you're dealing with – even the professionals can be unsure – do not just make a snap diagnosis. Instead respond only to those symptoms you understand, such as dehydration and respiratory problems, and deal with these while accepting you do not know the root cause. That is all that can be expected of you.

Glossary

ABC – stands for Airway, Breathing, Circulation, the primary vital signs checks.

Adrenaline – a hormone secreted by the adrenal glands to allow the body to meet conditions of stress.

Altitude sickness – illness resulting from oxygen deprivation at high altitudes.

Alveoli – tiny air sacs in the lungs through which gases are passed to and from the blood.

Amoebic dysentery – a chronic dehydrating illness resulting from an infection by microscopic amoebas.

Anaemia – a deficiency of haemoglobin or red blood cells in the blood resulting in fatigue and pale skin colour.

Anaphylaxis – a major allergic reaction resulting in generalized swelling and vascular shock.

Angina pectoris – a condition caused by narrowed coronary arteries which restrict blood flow to the heart, resulting in severe chest pains during times of exertion.

Antibiotic – a medicine that controls or destroys micro-organisms.

Antihistamine – a medicine that controls inflammatory reactions.

Antiseptic – chemicals which destroy micro-organisms and thus prevent disease.

Aorta – the main artery which supplies oxygenated blood to the body.

Appendicitis – inflammation and swelling of the appendix.

AR – an abbreviation for Artificial Respiration.

Arteries – the blood vessels through which oxygenated blood is transferred through the human body.

Asthma – an illness characterized by muscular spasms in the respiratory system and by a swelling of the airways.

Autonomic nervous system – the part of the nervous system concerned with involuntary nervous reactions and processes.

AVPU – a code used in checking levels of consciousness, standing for Alert, Voice, Pain, Unconscious.

Avulsion – a tearing or pulling injury.

Blister – a serum-filled bubble on the skin caused by an injury, usually heat or friction related.

Brainstem – a part of the brain which deals with major vital functions such as breathing and heart rate.

Bronchi – the major air passages of the lungs which branch out from the base of the windpipe, and which subdivide into the bronchioles.

Bronchitis – an illness caused by inflammation of mucous membranes in the bronchial tubes.

Bruise – an injury resulting from a blow to the skin which damages blood vessels.

Cardiogenic shock – shock resulting from ineffective heart action.

Cerebellum – the part of the brain responsible for control of movement and balance.

Cerebral compression – dangerous pressure placed on the brain through either a blood build-up in the skull or through a swelling of the brain itself.

Cerebrum – the large front part of the brain which, amongst other things, controls conscious thought and sensation.

Cholera – an infectious bacterial disease of the small intestine, usually spread through infected water, resulting in dehydration by severe vomiting and diarrhoea.

Circulatory system – the system which distributes blood throughout the human body, consisting of the heart and various blood vessels.

Closed fracture – a fracture which is contained within unbroken skin.

Comminuted fracture – a type of fracture which produces multiple bone fragments at the break site.

Concussion – unconsciousness, usually temporary, which results from a blow to the head.

Convulsion – any type of involuntary physical seizure or muscle spasm usually associated with brain disorders.

Core temperature – the temperature of the internal organs, ideally within the optimum range of 36–38°C (97.8–100°F).

CPR – an abbreviation of Cardio-Pulmonary Resuscitation.

Cyanosis – a bluing of the skin caused by a circulatory disorder reducing levels of oxygenated blood.

Dehydration – the loss of levels of water greater than the levels being introduced.

Dengue – a mosquito-transferred viral disease resulting in fever and severe joint pain.

Dermis – the layer of tissue beneath the outer skin which contains most of the skin's functioning elements such as nerve endings, sweat glands and blood capillaries.

Diabetes mellitus – the most prevalent form of diabetes which results from a deficiency of insulin and thus causes a lack of control over blood-sugar levels.

Diphtheria – an acute infectious bacterial disease which attacks respiration and can cause fatal heart and nerve damage.

Dislocation – the unseating of a body joint from its normal position.

Epidermis – the outermost layer of the skin.

Epilepsy – a disorder of the nervous system caused by disruptions of normal electrical activity in the brain, the result being seizures, convulsions and loss of consciousness.

Epinephrine – a synthetic form of adrenaline often used in the treatment of anaphylaxis.

Faint – a temporary loss of consciousness owing to a drop in blood pressure and a lack of oxygen to the brain.

Fibrillation – when in the heart, fibrillation implies a rapid spasm which results in an ineffective heart beat.

First degree burns – burns which only affect the surface layer of the skin.

Frostbite – an injury to body tissue which has been exposed to severe cold temperatures, resulting in localized freezing.

Glaucoma – an increased pressure within the eyeball which disturbs vision and can lead to loss of sight.

HACE – an abbreviation of High-Altitude Cerebral Edema, a typical form of altitude sickness which involves a swelling of the brain.

Haemoglobin – a protein in human blood responsible for the transportation of oxygen around the body.

Haemothorax – a gathering of blood in the chest cavity usually following an injury.

HAPE – an abbreviation of High-Altitude Pulmonary Edema, a form of altitude sickness.

Heart attack – a sudden coronary thrombosis which can result in the death of a section of heart muscle.

Heat exhaustion – shock caused by fluid loss through sweating in response to environmental high temperatures.

Heimlich manoeuvre – a technique of removing an object lodged in someone's windpipe by applying a sudden strong upward pressure to the abdomen just beneath the rib cage.

Hepatitis – a disease which causes inflammation of the liver.

Hernia – a disorder in which an organ protrudes through the cavity which is meant to contain it.

Hyperglaecemia – a blood-sugar disorder caused by an excess of glucose in the blood.

Hyperthermia – a condition in which the body's core temperature is raised dangerously above its optimum range.

Hyperventilation – to breathe with abnormal rapidity and thus evacuate too much carbon dioxide from the body.

Hypoglaecemia – inadequate quantities of glucose in the blood.

Hypothermia – a condition in which the body's core temperature drops dangerously below its optimum range.

Hypoxia – a condition caused by an inadequate amount of oxygen reaching body tissue through the blood stream.

Infarction – the cutting off of blood supply to a particular region of tissue which results in localized tissue death.

Insulin – a pancreatic hormone which regulates the amount of glucose in the blood.

Iritis – the inflammation of the iris of the eye.

Ischemia – an lack of effective blood supply to a particular region of the body.

Ligaments – the piece of connective tissue which holds two bones or a joint together.

Malaria – a disease transmitted by mosquitoes which results in a recurrent pattern of fever.

Meninges – the three membranes which enclose the brain and spinal cord.

Miliaria – a medical name for prickly heat.

Morphine – a drug extracted from opium and used medicinally in pain relief.

Nervous system – the body system consisting of the brain, spinal cord, peripheral nervous system and autonomic nervous system.

Open fracture – a fracture in which the broken bone has torn through the skin to be externally exposed.

Peripheral nervous system – the network of nerves which connect the spinal cord and brain with the rest of the body.

Peritonitis – the inflammation of the membrane which lines the abdominal cavity and covers the abdominal organs.

Pneumonia – a chronic lung infection which fills the lung's air sacs with puss.

Pneumothorax – the intrusion of air or gas between the lung and the chest wall the pressure of which can result in a collapsed lung.

Poliomyelitis – a viral disease which can produce various levels of analysis by attacking the central nervous system

Postural drainage – the technique of evacuation mucus or pus from the lungs by pounding the patient's back while they are in a head down position.

Respiratory system – the body system comprising the mouth, nose, trachea, lungs and pulmonary blood vessels.

Second degree burns – burns which have damaged several layers of the epidermis resulting in blistering and rawness.

Shock – an inefficient transfer of oxygen from the blood to the body tissue caused by injury to the circulatory and/or respiratory systems.

Simple fracture – a fracture in which the bone is broken cleanly.

Snow blindness – visual impairment caused by the reflective glare of the sun off snow.

Spinal cord – the cord of nerves and fibres which run through the spine and connects most of the body with the brain as part of the central nervous system.

Stable fracture – a fracture which results in the broken bones being jammed together in such a way as to make the limb or area relatively stable.

Sternum – the breastbone.

Stroke – a sudden impairment of blood flow to a region of the brain caused by either a haemorrhage or a blood clot.

Tendons – a strong collagen cord which attaches a muscle to a bone.

Tetanus – a disease caused by the ingress of bacteria which results in rigid and spasmodic muscles.

Third degree burns – burns which damage tissue to a depth below the skin.

Thrombosis – a localized blockage in the circulatory system caused by blood coagulation or clotting.

Trachea – a medical term for the windpipe.

Traction – the technique of aligning a fractured limb or relocating a dislocated joint by pulling on the limb and then releasing it into its normal position.

Tuberculosis – a bacterial disease, usually of the lungs, in which nodules grow on the affected tissue.

Typhoid – an infectious bacterial disease which results in fever, rash and dehydrating illnesses.

Typhus – the term for several types of disease with symptoms similar to typhoid; tends to be associated with insanitary conditions.

Unstable fracture – a fracture which results in an unstable relation of the broken pieces of bone to one another.

Vascular shock – a form of shock caused by a chronic dilation of the blood vessels.

Veins – blood vessels which mainly carry deoxygenated blood back to the heart.

Volume shock – shock created through the loss of fluid volume from the body.

Yellow fever – a tropical disease transmitted by mosquitoes which attacks the liver and the kidneys.

Survival kitbag contents

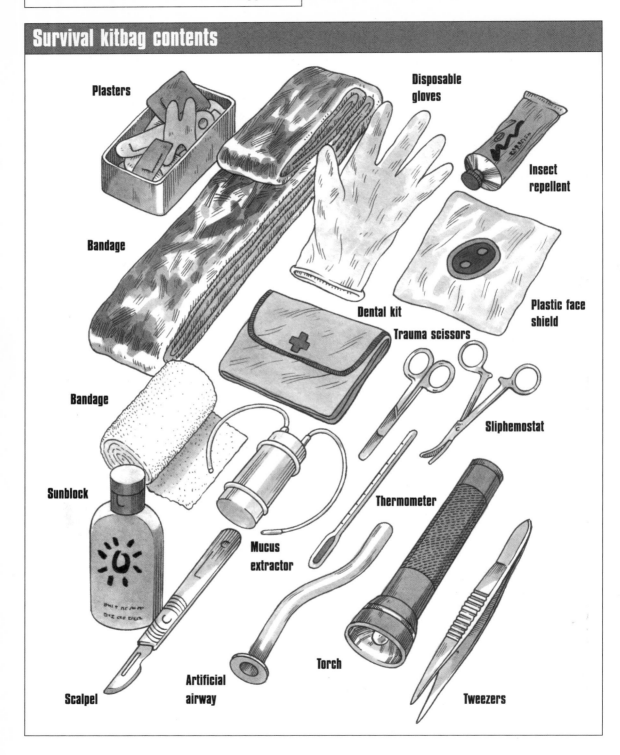

Plasters

Disposable gloves

Insect repellent

Bandage

Dental kit

Plastic face shield

Bandage

Trauma scissors

Sliphemostat

Sunblock

Thermometer

Mucus extractor

Scalpel

Artificial airway

Torch

Tweezers

Index